SpringerBriefs in Psychology

Behavioral Criminology

Series editor

Vincent B. Van Hasselt, Fort Lauderdale, USA

More information about this series at http://www.springer.com/series/10850

Charles J. Golden · Lucas D. Driskell
Lisa K. Lashley

The Intercorrelation of Traumatic Brain Injury and PTSD in Neuropsychological Evaluations

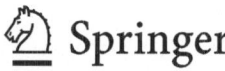 Springer

Charles J. Golden
Department of Psychology
Nova Southeastern University
Fort Lauderdale, FL
USA

Lisa K. Lashley
Nova Southeastern University
Fort Lauderdale, FL
USA

Lucas D. Driskell
College of Psychology
Nova Southeastern University
Fort Lauderdale, FL
USA

ISSN 2192-8363   ISSN 2192-8371   (electronic)
SpringerBriefs in Psychology
ISSN 2194-1866   ISSN 2194-1874   (electronic)
SpringerBriefs in Behavioral Criminology
ISBN 978-3-319-47032-0   ISBN 978-3-319-47033-7   (eBook)
DOI 10.1007/978-3-319-47033-7

Library of Congress Control Number: 2016953321

Printed on acid-free paper

This Springer imprint is published by Springer Nature
The registered company is Springer International Publishing AG
The registered company address is: Gewerbestrasse 11, 6330 Cham, Switzerland

Contents

Chapter 1
Introduction

Differential diagnosis of conditions with overlapping symptoms is critical in identifying the likely course and treatment for a client. This book attempts to provide a review of the neuropsychological science and clinical implications of the relationship between traumatic brain injury (TBI) and posttraumatic stress disorder (PTSD). Prior research has extensively explored the similarities between TBI and PTSD (Belanger et al. 2009; Bryant and Harvey 1998; Hoge et al. 2008; McMillan et al. 2003; Schneiderman et al. 2008; Warden 2006); however, there are still difficulties with the assessment, conceptualization, and treatment of the two disorders. This book was designed to offer those interested in TBI and PTSD a neuropsychological reference guide to aid in clinical decisions and supplement the current body of the literature on the respective disorders. To appeal to all audiences, first a brief review of the clinical neuropsychology profession is conducted.

The field of clinical neuropsychology is a specialty field that aims to develop a deeper understanding of the brain–behavior relationship, specifically for more accurate assessment, diagnoses of neurological and cognitive disorders, and treatment recommendations. In its very early years, the practice of clinical neuropsychology was composed of psychologists attempting to acquire what information they could from intelligence tests and possibly the Bender-Gestalt or Memory for Designs tests, in hopes of gaining insight into general brain dysfunction (Golden et al. 1992; Golden and Lashley 2014). It was not until Dr. Ward Halstead and one of his doctoral students, Ralph Reitan, developed and validated the Halstead-Reitan Battery (HRNB) that the purpose and results of neuropsychological assessment proved to be invaluable to the medical and psychological field.

The HRNB allowed neuropsychologist to evaluate a wide range of nervous system and brain functions, including verbal and auditory skills, spatial and sequential perception, motor skills, attention, concentration, expressive and receptive

© The Author(s) 2016
C.J. Golden et al., *The Intercorrelation of Traumatic Brain Injury and PTSD in Neuropsychological Evaluations*, SpringerBriefs in Behavioral Criminology, DOI 10.1007/978-3-319-47033-7_1

language, and executive functioning. During this time, the main purpose of neuro-psychological assessment was to determine if there was brain damage, and if so, where it is located. From the information obtained by the assessment's results, one may postulate the cognitive and emotional ramifications of the specific neurologic injury. However, over time the theory and focus behind neuropsychological assessment shifted from localization and etiology to a more comprehensive evaluation that strongly incorporates factors such as psychological health and history, environmental and familial resources, cognitive strengths and weaknesses, and personality characteristics.

Now the practice of neuropsychology encompasses a wide range of applications ranging from assistance in diagnostic and treatment of known or suspected central nervous system dysfunctions, the evaluation of effectiveness of pharmacologic and surgical therapies, and the differentiation of cognitive, personality, and neurological causes of presenting problems. Moreover, recently, neuropsychological evaluations have become pivotal in the forensic realm, providing the court with a deeper understanding of the behavioral, emotional, and cognitive consequences of a known or suspected central nervous system dysfunction. Golden (1976) foresaw the necessity and advantages of focusing on understanding the client from a cognitive and personality perspective utilizing a brain-behavior framework, rather than as a possible conclusion to derive.

The focus in the field has been mostly pointed towards the understanding and differentiation of different neurological disorders, with less attention to psychiatric disorders. Early in the career of the senior author, one major question was whether a disorder was either organic or psychiatric, suggesting that these were mutually exclusive categories. This question was most often generated by individuals whose schizophrenia or major depression was refractive to treatment, raising the question of whether they really had these disorders. Primarily cognitive testing assisted by the Minnesota Multiphasic Personality Inventory (MMPI) was used to see if cognitive skills fell into a "brain injury range" as defined by the theoretical and psychometric approaches of the clinician. With the advent of CT scans and subsequent improvements in neuroradiological evidence, it became increasingly evident that many people with serious mental disorders had evidence of structural damage to the brain. If one includes the role of neurotransmitters (as opposed to structural damage), then the percentage of individuals with neuropsychological problems and psychiatric symptoms increases substantially.

One impediment in the full exploration of these issues has been the focus of neuropsychologists on the cognitive rather than the emotional and behavioral effects of disorders. While the Diagnostic and Statistical Manuals (over all editions) have provided categories for emotional disorders caused by medical conditions (including neurological disorders), but such categories were and remain poorly defined and used inconsistently. As will be seen later in this book, the issues of whether a disorder is emotional (PTSD) or neuropsychological (TBI) may be clear in some cases; however, in many cases we may be talking about a joint disorder which has both emotional (environmental or experiential) roots along with a clear structural neuropsychological component (brain damage) as well as neurotransmission/neurotransmitter issues (brain dysfunction) may not fit either category clearly and may represent a new disorder or subtype not currently recognized or properly treated.

Cognitive capacity, personality, and brain functioning all play crucial roles in understanding the relationship between TBI and PTSD, as do the roles of the social and physical environment, personal history, and both emotional and physical trauma. The interplay of each of these will be addressed, beginning with a review of some of the relevant research in the next chapter.

Chapter 2
The Research

For years now the relationship between traumatic brain injuries (TBIs) and post-traumatic stress disorder (PTSD) has been a controversial issue that seems to leave many unanswered questions. The most salient issue is whether an individual with a TBI can develop PTSD if they have no memory of the incident. While they share many commonalities, such as symptomatology, and even more obvious ones, like the fact that they both stem from a traumatic event, not all traumatic events result in TBI or PTSD. Among individuals in the United States, approximately 61 % of men and 51 % of women will be exposed to trauma during their lifetime, but only about 5 % of men and 10 % of women will develop PTSD based on the National Comorbidity Survey (Kessler et al. 1995). It has been estimated that there are nearly 10 million TBI incidences annually, with almost 1.7 million emergency department visits yearly in the United States (Hyder et al. 2007).

Yurgil et al. (2014) found in a military sample that TBI during one's most recent deployment is the strongest predictor of post-deployment PTSD, even when accounting for pre-deployment symptoms, prior TBIs, and combat intensity. It has long been recognized that TBI and PTSD evidence many of the same symptoms, resulting from physiological, neurological, and psychological damage. Dating back to World War I, it has been noted that soldiers who were exposed to mortar attacks and grenade blasts began to experience psychological and neurological symptoms, which at the time was termed "Shell Shock". With the growth of research on these symptoms and their origin, we have now made distinctions between brain injury and PTSD; however, differentiation often still becomes grayed.

There can be difficulty when assessing someone who has received brain injury from a traumatic event because TBI and PTSD share numerous symptoms. There is always the possibility of PTSD being overlooked in someone who presents with mood or behavioral difficulties (McMillan et al. 2003). Similarly, TBI may be

© The Author(s) 2016
C.J. Golden et al., *The Intercorrelation of Traumatic Brain Injury and PTSD in Neuropsychological Evaluations*, SpringerBriefs in Behavioral Criminology, DOI 10.1007/978-3-319-47033-7_2

overlooked if a person does not evidence any neurological symptoms and only presents with psychological complaints. While the identification of moderate and severe brain injuries tend to be much more straightforward, mild TBI and PTSD can present similar symptoms such as irritability, sleep disturbance, memory disturbance, personality and mood changes, shortened patience, depression, hostility, and anxiety. To test the extent of PTSD and TBI comorbidity, Hoofien et al. (2001) tested 76 patients who received a TBI diagnosis an average of 14 years before the study and found that 14 % still met full diagnostic criteria for PTSD.

The ultimate purpose of a neuropsychological evaluation is to provide recommendations that will inform the patient what steps they should take to address their presenting problems. In order to give appropriate recommendations, the neuropsychologist must be accurate in their conceptualization and diagnostic capabilities; and, in the case of differentiating TBI from PTSD, they must have a deep working knowledge of the neurological and psychological underpinnings of both disorders. Thus, before we look at specific approaches to understanding a patient that presents with TBI/PTSD symptoms, it is first necessary to examine what research has shown about each disorder individually. To date, much of the epidemiological research on the relationship between TBI and PTSD has focused on the military population, due to the prevalence of exposure to physically and psychologically traumatic events. However, even with this limitation, there is still ample research on TBI and PTSD individually, providing the authors the opportunity to gather a selected sample of research to emphasize the important aspects of these two disorders.

Traumatic Brain Injury

Traumatic brain injury (TBI) is a form of acquired brain injury, typically caused by a sudden blow to skull or violent jerk of the head. TBIs often result in either: (1) direct damage to the neurons of the brain, and/or (2) shearing of neuronal axons that allow the brain to communicate within its self and with the rest of the body. Due to the intricate nature of the brain's organization, symptoms of TBI widely vary depending on severity, location, and duration of the damage. Having said that, some more common symptoms of TBI range from headaches, confusion, vomiting, sleep disturbances, depression, anxiety, impaired attention, fatigue, speech impairments, visual spatial deficits, vision impairments, memory deficits, personality changes, mood disorders, paralysis, to death. Approximately 57 million people worldwide have been hospitalized with one or more TBIs (Murray and Lopez 1996).

It was estimated that in 2009, 2.4 million hospital emergency department visits, hospitalizations, or deaths related to a TBI occurred in the United States (Faul and Coronado 2014). In 2006, approximately 5.3 million people were living with significant disabilities caused by TBI that inhibited their ability to return to prior levels of functioning (Langlois et al. 2006). According to the World Health Organization, TBI will surpass numerous diseases as the major cause of disability and death by the year 2020.

On a global scale, the primary cause of TBI is road traffic accidents (62 %), with violence (24 %) and falls (8 %) ranked as second and third (Hyder et al. 2007). These statistics are not incorporating the vast amount of those who receive some form of brain injury and do not seek treatment. Since every brain trauma incident is unique to its source of injury, the assessment and treatment of such disorders can be a complicated task. Thus, TBIs can be categorized into different classifications depending upon cause and severity in order to aid in specificity of diagnosis and treatment.

There are three overall severity classifications that TBIs can be placed into: mild, moderate, and severe. Now each level of severity will be discussed in further detail.

Mild Traumatic Brain Injury. Mild TBI is described as neurological damage ranging from minimal to no change of severity from a patients usual cognition level (Bruns and Jagoda 2009). Prior research has found that mild TBIs substantially outnumber moderate and severe TBIs, accounting for an estimated 80 % of all TBIs (Elder et al. 2010; Hoge et al. 2008; Tanielian and Jaycox 2008). Bruns and Jagoda (2009) reported that only 1 % of mild TBIs will require neurosurgical intervention. While most people that receive a mild TBI recover relatively quickly and fully, this type of injury must not be overlooked. Mild TBI can still cause permanent neurological and neuropsychological dysfunction. Unfortunately, many people who receive mild TBI do not seek medical treatment because they are oblivious of the severity of their injury.

Currently, there is not one definitive definition of mild TBI because brain trauma is such an individualized-injury; however, the three most commonly used definitions of mild TBI were developed by: (1) the World Health Organization Collaborating Centre Task Force on Mild Traumatic Brain Injury in 2004, (2) the Center for Disease Control working group in 2003, and (3) the Mild Traumatic Brain Injury Committee of the Head Injury Interdisciplinary Special Interest Group of the American Congress of Rehabilitation Medicine in 1993. While all three definitions are slightly different from one another, they correspond on the majority of criteria. When integrated, the salient criteria for mild TBI are the patient having received an injury to the head from an external force or acceleration/deceleration forces that resulted in *one or more* of the following: confusion, disorientation, loss of consciousness for less than 30 min, dysfunction of memory around the time of injury, or observable neurological or neuropsychological dysfunction such as seizures or focal deficits.

In addition to the three definitions that were just discussed, the Glasgow Coma Scale (GCS) is almost always used in order to assess the severity of brain injury. The GCS ranks patients upon a neurological scale ranging from 3 to 15. A score of 13 or higher would classify as mild head trauma injury. A score ranging from 9 to 12 would classify as moderate head trauma injury, and any score of 8 or lower would fall in the range of severe head trauma. The scale is broken up into three dimensions: (1) stimulus required for eye opening, with a possible score of 1–4, (2) best verbal response, with a possible score of 1–5, and (3) best motor response, with a possible score of 1–6.

Many medical and psychological professionals recognize two subtypes of mild TBI: complicated and uncomplicated. Complicated mild TBI is diagnosed when the patient meets criteria for a mild TBI and has a brain abnormality (e.g., edema, hematoma, or contusion) visible on neuroimaging on the day of the injury (Iverson and Lange 2011). Conversely, uncomplicated mild TBI is diagnosed when the patient meets criteria for mild TBI, but does not evidence any damage via neuroimaging.

During the first few days after a mild TBI, many individuals report experiencing headaches, drowsiness, difficulty with concentration and attention, dizziness, and feeling mentally cloudy. These symptoms often last for days to weeks. There has been much discussion on determining factors that can predict neuropsychological outcome in patients with mild TBI. The two most researched factors are duration of loss of consciousness (LOC) and duration of posttraumatic amnesia (PTA). The term loss of consciousness is typically defined as a sleep-like state of being. Posttraumatic amnesia refers to the patient's inability to remember things that have happened immediately after the head trauma. As discussed by Iverson and Lange (2011), numerous researchers have reported that while there is no clear association between brief LOC and neuropsychological functioning (Leininger et al. 1990; Lovell et al. 1999), there appears to be a relationship between the presence and duration of PTA and worse immediate outcome and recovery (Collins et al. 2003; McCrea et al. 2002). In regards to neuropsychological performance after mild TBI, impairment in processing speed, working memory, verbal fluency, executive functioning, new learning, and memory are most commonly seen (Alexander 1995; Barrow et al. 2006; Belanger et al. 2005; McAllister et al. 2006).

Moderate and Severe Traumatic Brain Injury. While mild TBIs account for the majority of brain injuries (80 %), moderate (10 %) and severe (10 %) brain injuries are estimated to evenly comprise the rest of the distribution. Similarly to mild TBI, there is no one definitive definition for moderate or severe TBIs; thus, the GCS, duration of LOC, and duration of PTA are most often used for differentiation and diagnosis. For moderate TBI, many abide by the criteria of a GCS ranging from 9 to 12, duration of LOC of 30 min to 24 h, and duration of PTA of 1–7 days. For severe TBI GCS of 3–8, duration of LOC of more than 24 h, and duration of PTA greater than 7 days is most commonly used.

Moderate TBI is similar to mild TBI in the sense that it may go undiagnosed because the victim does not seek medical assistance. Moderate TBI symptoms are sometimes not as obvious as those of severe TBI. Many of those with moderate TBI seek treatment weeks to months after the incident with the concern of not feeling quite like himself or herself (Zillmer and Spiers 2001). A common complaint of both moderate and severe TBI is memory disruption. As already mentioned, many individuals experience PTA (also known as anterograde amnesia) and have difficulty remembering events that have occurred after their head trauma. Depending on numerous factors, symptoms of PTA can last from minutes to months. On the contrary, the inability to remember events that occurred before a head trauma is commonly referred to as retrograde amnesia. Similarly to PTA, retrograde amnesia ranges in duration of memory impairment and the date to which the individual can remember (e.g., whether one week or three years prior to the head trauma).

Along with classifications of severity, there are also classifications of injury processes in the brain. Moderate and severe TBI can both present with major complications such as edema of the brain, intracranial bleeding, skull fractures, and brain herniation. Primary injury in TBI occurs at the moment of the trauma and is a direct result of the injury. Common primary brain injuries are hemorrhages, contusions, concussions, and axonal fiber ripping. Secondary brain injury is damage that may be caused by a primary injury. It is important to note that secondary brain injury is an indirect result of the primary injury. Secondary brain injuries may appear days, weeks, or months after the primary injury. Secondary brain injuries may present as edema, increased intracranial pressure, intracranial infection, necrosis, apoptosis, or epilepsy. When assessing the extent to which one with severe TBI will recover, the severity of primary brain injury and the development of secondary brain damage are crucial deciding factors.

Closed and Penetrating Head Injuries. Physical damage to the brain can result from two methods of injury, either an object penetrating the skull and damaging the brain, or the rapid acceleration and/or deceleration of the head causing the brain to hit the insides of the skull. These mechanisms of physical brain injury are separated into two classifications, penetrating and closed head injuries. Penetrating head injuries occur when fractures the skull and damages specific regions of the brain. The resulting symptoms are dependent upon the localization of damage and complications with infections or hemorrhaging. In some cases, the fracturing of the skull can actually protect the brain by absorbing the force of the blow and not transmitting it into the brain itself as seen in closed head injuries.

Closed head injuries are the result of the brain undergoing acceleration and/or deceleration. When the brain endures acceleration, the head rapidly changes from stationary to moving causing the stationary brain to smash into the moving cranium. An example of acceleration would be a person's head being hit by an object such as a tree limb or baseball bat. Deceleration of the brain would occur when the head is moving at a constant speed, but then is stopped abruptly. An example would be an individual riding in a car that is forced to slam on its brakes, causing the person to fly forward and slam their head upon the windshield. Although the person's head would immediately stop once it hit the windshield, the brain floating in cerebral spinal fluid would slam into the front of the skull close to the same speed the car was originally going. Both acceleration and deceleration can cause massive damage to the brain by ripping neuronal fibers, and bruising the brain from impact against the skull. Contusions can become very dangerous, resulting in hemorrhage and edema of the brain.

In some cases, closed head injuries result in a coup countercoup injury. The coup injury is the result of either the primary acceleration or deceleration, causing the brain to collide with the skull. The contrecoup occurs after the brain bounces off the skull from the first collision, and then hits the opposing side of the skull. Coup and contrecoup injuries can result in both focal and diffuse injuries, contusions, concussions, and the tearing of neuronal fibers.

There are several caveats to these classifications. In some cases, a closed-head injury may cause focal damage because of a vascular tear or rupture which causes focal bleeding in the brain. Such bleeding can result in hematomas, often in the subdural area of the brain. In these cases, the hematoma will grow and become a mass which acts like a space occupying lesion. If treated quickly or if it resolves spontaneously, such hematomas while sounding scary may have no impact. However, when not treated they can continue to grow to a size where the internal pressure of the brain is raised, causing damage to tissue and even cutting off blood flow to the brain (as the heart cannot pump strongly enough to overcome the increased pressure) leading to anoxia or hypoxia and significant cognitive impairment or even death. While such disorders are more likely as we age, they can occur in anyone at any age.

A second but similar issue occurs when the bleedings occurs not in the meninges but within the grain itself as a result of a rupture of a blood vessel which may be related to the presence of a preexisting malformation or aneurysm. In such cases, bleeding may damage brain tissue and create a focal injury similar to that seen in penetrating injuries. Severity of the problems can range from mild to severe (even causing death) depending on many individual factors. Bleeding in the brain may of course also occur in penetrating head injuries.

Blast-Related Brain Injuries. Blast-related brain injuries become increasingly recognized by the military (rather than dismissing such disorders as emotional as has been done throughout history) as well as my the public after well publicized terrorist blast effects. It has been reported that the most common cause of war injuries are from explosions and blasts (Warden 2006). At the Walter Reed Army Medical Center, 59 % of patients who were tested for brain injury due to blast exposure were diagnosed with TBI (Okie 2005). Explosions pose as a serious threat to soldiers because of the many ways in which they can cause harm. There are four categories of blasts effects that are designated by the way a blast can cause injury. The first is primary (caused from pressure change), second is secondary (caused from projectiles), third is tertiary (caused from wind propelling the individual), and the fourth is quaternary (caused from burns, asphyxia, and toxin exposure) (DePalma et al. 2005).

Primary. Primary blast injuries consist of damage to the brain caused by the change of atmospheric pressure after an explosion. Once the explosion has occurred, there is a dramatic increase in atmospheric pressure caused by the oscillation of the blast waves. This rapid push of air from the explosion (increase of pressure) subsequently causes a vacuum effect, making the atmospheric pressure less than the norm. Then the second wave hits, causing the atmospheric pressure to increase slightly above the norm, before it then returns to a balanced pressure. For many years, this pressure change was believed to only harm the lungs, gastrointestinal tract, and the eardrums. However recently it has been argued that, primary blast injuries to the brain include concussion as well as barotrauma caused by acute gas embolism (DePalma et al. 2005). Although still controversial, primary blasts are believed by many to also harm the central nervous system.

Secondary and Tertiary. Secondary and tertiary blast injuries are the injuries most commonly thought of when one thinks of explosions. Blast waves propel shrapnel, foreign objects, and in many cases soldiers, in all directions. As a result, everyone in the vicinity becomes a target. Secondary blast injuries are those obtained by soldiers due to the undirected projection of foreign objects and shrapnel. In regards to the brain injury, secondary blast injuries can consist of both closed head and penetrating head injuries. Depending on how close someone is to the explosion, if they are wearing a helmet, the speed of the object being flung, and the shape of the object, dictates whether the injury will be closed head or penetrating. Tertiary blast injuries are sustained from the soldier being projected as an object due to the immense force of the blast wind. Soldiers are at high risk of both closed and penetrating head injuries when hurled by blast winds. In both secondary and tertiary blast injuries, the rapid acceleration and/or deceleration of the head can cause neuronal fiber tears, concussions, and contusions.

With the advancement of technology, IEDs and mortars have become extremely sophisticated. IEDs can be set off with a remote detonation, rigged for timed explosion, and even ignited by pressure sensors from vehicles driving above. In many cases, with the combination of bodily injury and psychological trauma caused by an explosion, many soldiers are unaware of the brain injury they received. Researchers believe that more than 30 % of troops who serve in active combat zones for four months or longer will receive neurological damage from IED and mortar blast waves, while presenting no surface damage (Glasser 2007). Trudeau et al. (1998) reported finding a subgroup of patients with PTSD who, although they had a history of mild concussion on exposure to explosions, had never been diagnosed with brain injury. There is still little known about the neuropsychological ramifications of blast induced brain trauma, making the differentiation between PTSD and TBI more difficult to determine.

Quatenary. Quaternary effects are caused by indirect effects caused from burns, respiratory difficulties causing hypoxia and anoxia, cardiac arrest, exposure to toxins, excessive blood lost, and injuries to other bodily systems. This is clearly difficult to define as the possibilities are nearly endless and depend on the exact factor in each individual situation. In many cases, the individual will die or suffer such extreme disabilities that neuropsychological testing will never take place, but in other cases these factors can cause extreme cognitive and emotional problems arising from brain damage or secondary injury, as well as the emotional effects of such events.

Common Psychological Outcomes of Traumatic Brain Injuries. Traumatic brain injuries often result in psychological symptoms and disorders. One of the most famous examples of the brain's role in personality is the case of Phineas Gage, a railroad worker who survived an accident during which an iron rod went straight through his left frontal lobe. Before his accident Phineas Gage was described as a hard working, responsible, and pleasant man; however, after the accident he was seen to be fitful, impulsive, and disrespectful. The case of Phineas Gage ignited the field of research on the relationship between the brain and psychological disorders, and while leaps and bounds have been made since his accident, there is still much to discover.

Some of the most common psychological disorders associated with TBIs are major depression, generalized anxiety disorder, PTSD, panic disorder, obsessive–compulsive disorder, substance abuse, and specific phobia (Deb et al. 1999; Federoff et al. 1992; Hibbard et al. 1998; Jorge et al. 1993; Van Reekum et al. 1996). Within the literature there are vast differences in reported post-TBI rates of psychological disorders. In regards to major depression, the prevalence rate ranges from 14–77 % depending on the study at which one looks (Deb et al. 1999; Fann et al. 1995; Federoff et al. 1992; Hibbard et al. 1998; Jorge et al. 1993; Van Reekum et al. 1996; Varney et al. 1987). Various studies report rates of 3–28 % for generalized anxiety disorder (Fann et al. 1995; Hibbard et al. 1998; Jorge et al. 1993; Van Reekum et al. 1996), and 3–27 % for PTSD (Bryant et al. 2000; Deb et al. 1999; Hibbard et al. 1998). Moreover, 4–17 % receives a diagnosis of panic disorder, 2–15 % receive obsessive–compulsive disorder, and 1–10 % received phobic disorder diagnosis, while 5–28 % receive a diagnosis of substance abuse (Deb et al. 1999; Hibbard et al. 1998; Van Reekum et al. 1996).

In attempt to determine the long-term effects of TBI on psychological health, Koponen et al. (2002) evaluated 60 patients on an average of 30 years after their TBI. The Schedules for Clinical Assessment in Neuropsychiatry was used to help assess the Axis I disorders, while the Structured Clinical Interview for DSM-III-R Personality Disorders was utilized for the Axis II disorders. The researchers found that 61.7 % of patients had an Axis I disorder during their lifetimes, and 40 % had an Axis I disorder at the time of evaluation. Of the 60 patients, 48 % had an Axis I disorder develop after the TBI, while 22 % had an Axis I disorder before their TBI. The most common Axis I disorder found post-TBI was major depression, occurring in 27 % of patients at some point after the TBI, and 10 % at the time of assessment. Panic disorder was diagnosed in 8 % of patients at some point after the TBI, and 7 % still met criteria for panic disorder. 12 % of the male patients met criteria for a substance abuse disorder after their TBI, while 8 % had the disorder at the time of assessment. 23 % of the patients had at least one personality disorder after their TBI, 15 % were avoidant, 8 % were paranoid, and 7 % were schizoid. The findings of this study suggests that, not only can TBI cause psychiatric disorders, but the effects of TBI on psychological health can be long-lasting, in many cases lasting longer than 30 years. In particular, TBI seems to be a major risk factor for disorders, such as major depression, substance abuse, and the development of various personality disorders.

While there is a plethora of research on psychological outcomes of TBI, there tends to be numerous problems that researchers run into when attempting to study this phenomenon. First, a common methodological problem is that most studies do not take into account is that individuals with TBI tend to have difficulty with retrospective reporting of issues before their TBI. Being that one of the strongest predictors of psychological illness is prior psychological illness, this leads one to question the validity in results of psychological illnesses resulting from TBI. Second, some studies only look at the presenting disorder at the time of the study, which may be 1–30 years after the TBI, rather than looking at the whole history of psychological problems. This large range in time also makes it difficult to understand a timeline and progression of psychological problems after a TBI.

In order to address some of these concerns, Ashman et al. (2004) conducted a longitudinal study and a simultaneous cross-sectional study to examine the frequency of Axis I disorders in persons with TBI during the first 6 years post-injury. At the Research and Training Center in the Department of Rehabilitation and Medicine at

Mount Sinai School of Medicine in New York City, 188 participants that had received a TBI within the previous four years were recruited. Participants completed either two or three assessments, each one-year apart from each other. The semi-structured clinical interview called the Structured Clinical Interview for the Diagnostic and Statistical Manual of Mental Disorders, 4th Edition was utilized in order to assist clinicians in diagnostic accuracy. Of the 188 participants, 29 % have mild TBI, 62 % had moderate or severe TBI, and 9 % had loss of consciousness of unknown duration. One important finding from this study was that there were few cross-sectional differences in age; thus, age at the time of injury had little impact on Axis I diagnoses. In regards to gender, significantly more women met criteria for PTSD, depression, and anxiety disorder after their TBI than men. However, significantly more men met criteria for a substance abuse disorder. Also, the researchers found that psychological disorders pre-injury significantly predicted the presence of post-injury diagnosis. When controlling for this factor there was still a significant frequency of depression, PTSD, and anxiety post-TBI. Overall, the results of the study indicated that: (1) there is a high frequency of individuals that develop an Axis I disorder after TBI, and (2) there is an inverse relationship between odds of developing an Axis I disorder after TBI and time since injury, meaning your chances of having an Axis I disorder after a TBI declines over time.

Posttraumatic Stress Disorder

The Diagnostic and Statistical Manual, fifth edition (DSM-5) characterizes Posttraumatic Stress Disorder (PTSD) by the development of distinct symptoms after exposure to one or more traumatic events. Exposure can consist of directly experiencing the event, witnessing a traumatic event, learning about traumatic events that have happened to loved ones, and being exposed to the aftermath of traumatic events. Another feature of PTSD is the presence of intrusive symptoms, such as nightmares, flashbacks, or marked physiological reactions to internal or external cues that remind the person of the trauma. Persistent avoidance of such cues and familiar stimuli, as well as marked changes in cognition and arousal are typically present. Changes in cognition may present as difficulty with memory, distortions about the cause or consequences of the traumatic event, fear, horror, anger, diminished interests, and inability to experience positive emotions (American Psychiatric Association 2013). Alterations in arousal and reactivity often present as irritability, anger outburst, recklessness, hypervigilance, problems with concentration, and sleep disturbances (American Psychiatric Association 2013).

Although this is just one disorder, the clinical presentation can vary. While some individuals with PTSD present predominately with a depressed mood and negative cognitions, others are characterized by a more fear-based, behavioral and emotional reaction (American Psychiatric Association 2013). In others, hypervigilance and arousal are predominant, while in some a more dissociative reaction is present (American Psychiatric Association 2013). Neuropsychologically speaking, PTSD has been shown to cause significant impairments in memory, learning, attention, and executive functioning (Johnsen and Asbjørnsen 2008; Vasterling et al. 1998; Yehuda et al. 2004).

The DSM-5 reports that the lifetime risk of developing PTSD in the United States is 8.7 %, and the 12-month prevalence among adults is 3.5 % (2013). Not surprisingly so, an estimated one-third to more than one-half of those who are survivors of rape, military combat and captivity, and political or cultural internment and genocide develop PTSD. This disorder appears to be less prevalent in young children and older adults who are exposed to a traumatic event.

Acute Stress Disorder. While the main focus of this book is PTSD and TBI, an explanation of acute stress disorder is warranted due to its strong predictive power of PTSD. Acute stress disorder is essentially the same disorder with the same symptom presentation as PTSD, however, the key difference is the timeline. Acute stress disorder is diagnosed when the symptoms are present 3 days to 1 month after exposure to the traumatic event(s), whereas PTSD is diagnosed when the symptoms persist for more than 1 month. In order to investigate the relationship between acute stress disorder and PTSD, Harvey and Bryant (1998) assessed 92 motor vehicle accident survivors for acute stress disorder within 1 month of their trauma, and again at 6 months post-trauma for PTSD. After the first round of assessments within 1 month, 13 % of participants were diagnosed with acute stress disorder and 21 % had subclinical levels. At the 6-month follow-up, 78 % of the acute stress disorder patients and 60 % of the subclinical patients met criteria for PTSD. Specifically, the symptoms that had the strongest predictive power were acute numbing, depersonalization, sense of reliving the trauma, and motor restlessness. Countless studies since Harvey and Bryant's has supported the strong relationship between acute stress disorder and PTSD, and with the changes to both disorders in the latest DSM-5, the relationship appears to be stronger than before.

Neurocircuitry of Posttraumatic Stress Disorder. A unique feature of PTSD in comparison to most other psychiatric disorders is that the etiology is almost always well defined. Having such a specific cause helps neuroanatomical and neuropathological research, allowing researchers over the past few decades to use neuroimaging to test neurocircuitry hypotheses. To date, the strongest neurocircuitry model for PTSD is the fear-conditioning model. This model is based off of the three types of symptoms that characterize PTSD: (1) reexperiencing (flashbacks, nightmares, and physical pains), (2) avoidance (avoiding things that are reminders of the trauma, feeling numb, and losing interests in people and activities), and (3) hyperarousal (hypervigilance, easily startled, tension, emotionally labile, and difficulty sleeping). By connecting these symptoms with what is known about specific regions of the brain, it was determined that the limbic system, a region that plays a large role in emotional processing, appears to be involved in PTSD. Specifically within the limbic system, the brain structures implemented in PTSD are the prefrontal cortex (PFC), amygdala, and the hippocampus. The PFC is considered to be the brain region responsible for decision-making, personality, complex behavior, and social behavior. The amygdala, the control center for the fight-or-flight response, plays a key role in the learning and memory of fear responses. The hippocampus is best known as the region of the brain for short-term and long-term memory storage. After exposure to trauma, those with PTSD evidence reduced activation in the PFC and hippocampus, allowing the amygdala to over-respond to any potentially fearful events. The hyperresponsivity of the amygdala causes the strong emotional tie with the memory of the traumatic event, the under-activation of the PFC prevents the suppression of attention to trauma-related stimuli, and reduced hippocampal functioning causes the difficulties with the identification of safe stimuli and accompanying explicit memory difficulties (Bremner et al. 1995; Rauch et al. 2006).

Relationship Between TBI and PTSD

The acknowledgment that there is some form of relationship between TBI and PTSD, whether intentional or not, has been noted throughout history. Dating back to World War I, soldiers who were frequently exposed to mortar attacks and grenade blasts while fighting in the trenches were often diagnosed as having "Shell Shock". Shell Shock was a disorder characterized by amnesia, headaches, dizziness, tremors, and hypersensitivity. While such symptoms would typically be seen after a mild TBI, these soldiers evidenced no visual signs of head injuries. At the time, due to a lack of knowledge, doctors from all over disagreed on the cause of these symptoms. Some doctors posed that the soldiers had a hidden brain injury caused by the blast waves, while others argued the symptoms were due to carbon monoxide poisoning formed by the explosions. However, slowly overtime, doctors started to see soldiers with Shell Shock symptoms that were never exposed to explosions or mortar attacks; thus, the idea of a psychological cause was formed.

With the growth of research we have now made many distinctions between brain injury and psychological damage. However, the prevalence of comorbidity, as well as the difficulty of distinction between the correct origins of symptoms denotes the necessity for deeper understanding of the brain-behavior relationship in individuals with such disorders.

One of the first articles written to describe the occurrence of PTSD after a TBI was done so by McMillan (1991), in which he described the case of an 18-year-old female who was involved in a car wreck that resulted in a severe brain trauma and the death of her passenger. It was reported that she lost consciousness for at least three days. Initially the she suffered from mild right hemiparesis, mild dysphasia, euphoria, memory difficulties, and little insight. However, with rehabilitation, she made a strong recovery and returned to work after seven months. Fourteen months after the accident she returned complaining of fatigue, difficulty with concentration and coping at work, and some dizziness and severe headaches. Additionally, she expressed feelings of depression, failure, loss of interests, poor appetite, and hopelessness, obtaining a score of 27 (moderately severe range) on the Beck Depression Inventory (BDI). She was described by her mother to be irritable, verbally aggressive, and moody.

The patient reported having frequent intrusive thoughts of her dead friend throughout the day, as well as survivor guilt and strong anxiety when she thought about the wreck or when she entered a hospital. Along with other symptoms, she met full criteria for PTSD, while having a moderate degree of general impairment evidenced by neuropsychological testing 14 months after the wreck. After 4 months of therapy her BDI score fell to a 9 (not depressed), and her symptoms improved dramatically. This article serves as one of the first case studies to report in-depth that PTSD can develop despite experiencing a loss of consciousness. Moreover, that treatment for PTSD symptoms in an individual with TBI can prove to be efficacious.

In controversial study conducted by Sbordone and Liter (1995), the authors stated that it is highly unlikely that mild TBI patients actually develop PTSD symptoms. They examined 70 patients who had a previous diagnosis of either PTSD or mild TBI, and asked them to, in the most detail as possible, describe the traumatic event and the symptoms they developed from said event. The researchers found that while all of the patients with PTSD could provide a very detailed and emotionally charged recollection, none of those with mild TBI could. Moreover, none of the mild TBI patients reported any symptoms of intrusive thoughts, nightmares, hypervigilance, or startle reactions, nor did they become upset while talking about their traumatic event.

One of the first major studies to look at the neuropsychological relationship between PTSD and TBI was conducted by Hickling et al. (1998). Fueled by the desire to clear up the controversy as to whether one can actually develop PTSD after experiencing a TBI with loss of consciousness, the researchers attempted to answer two questions. First, they sought to determine whether motor vehicle accident (MVA) survivors who reported a loss of consciousness during their accident actually have lower rates of PTSD than those with no loss of consciousness. Second, the researchers posed if what is being called PTSD actually is due to brain injury, then those who meet criteria for PTSD should perform more poorly on neuropsychological testing; thus, they wanted to examine if those diagnosed with PTSD have greater neuropsychological dysfunction than those without PTSD in a brain-injured population. Of the 107 MVA survivors, 38 were diagnosed with PTSD. The researchers found that 40 % of those injured badly enough to lose consciousness met criteria for PTSD. Additionally, there were no differences found on neuropsychological testing between those who met criteria for PTSD and those who did not. Thus, this study suggests that many symptoms that are often attributed to PTSD may actually reflect the effects of TBI.

Bryant and Harvey (1998) conducted a study to determine if the occurrence of acute stress disorder following a mild TBI could be used to predict the development of PTSD. The researchers recruited 79 motor vehicle accident patients that sustained mild TBIs and tracked them for 6 months. Within 1 month of their injury patients were assessed for acute stress disorder, and after 6 months were assessed for PTSD using the PTSD module of the Composite International Diagnostic Interview. Acute stress disorder was diagnosed in 14 % of patients at 1 month, and at the 6-month follow-up 24 % satisfied criteria for PTSD. Of those diagnosed with acute stress disorder, 82 % were ultimately diagnosed with PTSD. Interestingly though, PTSD was diagnosed in 11 % of those who had not been diagnosed with acute stress disorder. This study provided two important findings, (1) PTSD after mild TBI is definitely a concern that should be addressed, and (2) acute stress disorder, although a strong predictor, does not always precede PTSD. In addition to these findings the authors discussed two important topics. First, diagnosing acute stress disorder after TBI could possibly be problematic because of the similarity and overlap of symptoms with postconcussive symptoms. Both acute stress disorder and postconcussive symptoms can present as derealization, depersonalization, and amnesia. Second, the authors point out that their frequency of PTSD with a TBI (24 %) after a motor vehicle accident is consistent to another study's finding of PTSD after a motor vehicle accident with no TBI (39 %; Blanchard et al. 1996), supporting that TBI does not impact the formation of PTSD.

Two years after their motor vehicle accident, Harvey and Bryant (2000) attempted to contact the original 79 patients for a follow-up evaluation, at which time 50 patients were willing to participate in the study. At the 2-year assessment, 22 % of the patients met criteria for PTSD. It was found that 80 % of the patients originally diagnosed with acute stress disorder met criteria for PTSD after 2 years. Interestingly, of those who were originally not diagnosed with acute stress disorder, 8 % met criteria for PTSD.

After investigating if PTSD could develop after mild TBI, Bryant et al. (2000) sought to determine if PTSD could occur after severe TBI. They utilized the theory that postulates the conditioned fear of trauma is mediated in subcortical regions of the brain rather than in higher cortical processes, suggesting that even when severe brain injury (which is typically cortical) occurs, one is still able to reexperience the trauma. Bryant and colleagues predicted that those who develop PTSD after severe TBI would have trauma reexperiencing in the form of emotional and physiological reactivity instead of intrusive memories.

The researchers assessed 96 severely brain-injured patients 6 months after their injury and found that 27 % met criteria for PTSD. Upon further analysis they found that only 19.2 % of the patients with PTSD reported intrusive memories of the trauma, while 96.2 % reported emotional reactivity and 50 % reported physiological reactivity. Specifically, symptoms, such as intrusive memories, nightmares, and emotional reactivity, were found to have very strong positive predictive powers for the development of PTSD. These findings support their theory that first, PTSD can develop after severe brain injury, and second, trauma reexperiencing can be mediated by fear conditioning or mental representations rather than explicit memories.

Williams et al. (2002) also investigated the prevalence of PTSD symptoms after severe TBI. The authors utilized a community sample of 66 individuals, 51 of which had been involved in road accidents (30 as drivers, 11 as passengers, 7 as pedestrians, 3 as cyclists), 12 suffered falls, 2 were physically assaulted, and 1 was involved in a bomb explosion. The sample varied significantly with a range of 1–26 years since their traumatic event, age range of 17–70 years of age, and an education range of 9–19 years. Duration of loss of consciousness and posttraumatic amnesia were used to determine TBI severity level. The overall finding was that 18 % of their community sample had PTSD symptoms, of which 6 % had severe symptoms. It is important to note that this finding is lower than what was found by Hickling et al. (1998) in individuals with mild TBI, suggesting that more severe the brain injury is, the less likely one is to develop PTSD afterwards.

While it was becoming supported that TBI and PTSD can co-occur, Van Reekum et al. (2000) sought to determine if there is a causative relationship between TBI and psychiatric disorders. The authors point out that if a causative relationship is found, it will have major implications for preventative measures after TBI, as well as litigation outcomes. Often it is the case that neuropsychologists are determining if someone's post-TBI difficulties are due to their TBI or due to a psychiatric disorder, as if they are separate. However, if there were a causative relationship, then one's problems would be secondary to psychiatric disorder, which is secondary to the TBI. Reekum and colleagues conducted a literature review on 42 articles, looking at disorders such as Depression, Bipolar, Generalized Anxiety Disorder, Obsessive–Compulsive Disorder, Panic Disorder, PTSD, Schizophrenia, Substance Abuse, and Personality Disorders. While there was strong evidence that TBI frequently caused some psychiatric disorders (Depression, Bipolar, Anxiety Disorders), there was no evidence that TBI caused PTSD. Actually, the findings suggested an inverse relationship between TBI and PTSD, in that PTSD is more common amongst mild TBI than it is amongst moderate or severe TBI, supporting the statement made by Williams et al. (2002). The authors raise the point that more severe TBI may be a protective factor for some psychiatric disorders due to sequelae such as reduced insight.

Bombardier et al. (2006) recognized that while numerous studies have looked at the prevalence rate for PTSD after TBI, very few have investigated if factors found to be predictive of PTSD in other patient populations increase the risk of developing PTSD in a TBI population. Predictors such as being female, little education, history of anxiety or depression, less severe brain injury, being assaulted, strong emotional reactions to the incident, and being under the influence of stimulant drugs. Another main question to their study was to what extent is meeting symptom criteria for PTSD associated with other current or past psychiatric disorders. Patients were recruited from a hospital in Seattle, Washington, and were determined to have a TBI by either radiological evidence of acute brain abnormality or a GCS score less than or equal to 12 within the first 24 h of admission. Over the course of 6 months, 125 participants were administered the 17-item PTSD Checklist-Civilian Version (PCL-C), the depression, panic, and anxiety modules of the Patient Health Questionnaire (PHQ), the one-item General Heath Scale from the SF-36, as well as a interview inquiring about history, demographic data, and medical variables.

The authors found that in their sample of complicated mild to severe TBI, 11.3 % met PTSD symptom criteria. They also found that those with more severe TBI had a lower incidence of PTSD than those with milder TBI. The authors point out that the incidence of PTSD after TBI from a motor vehicle accident is much lower than PTSD after a motor vehicle accident with no TBI, which is at least 34 % (Blanchard et al. 1995; Ursano et al. 1999). In regards to factors that contribute to the diagnosis of PTSD, the researchers found that people with less than a high school education were at a higher risk than those with more education. Also, those who recall feeling terrified or helpless, as well as those that were assaulted, were more likely to meet criteria for PTSD. Lastly, those who had used stimulant drugs (such as cocaine or amphetamine) around the time of trauma were more likely to develop PTSD. Interestingly, while meeting criteria for PTSD was significantly related to greater psychosocial impairment, it was not related to poorer subjective health ratings. However, the authors only using one question to measure subjective health may have limited this. Probably the most salient issued raised by this study is the necessity of assessing past and current psychological history. The authors reported that 29 % of those who met PTSD symptom criteria reported a having a history of PTSD before the accident. Thus, PTSD symptoms after a TBI may really just be a continuation or exacerbation of the individual's previous diagnoses. Additionally, it was remarkable that 79 % of those who met PTSD symptom criteria also reported symptoms consistent with major depressive disorder. Moreover, 71 % of those that met PTSD symptom criteria reported having major depressive disorder before their injury. Thus it is suggested that depression may play a large role as a risk factor for PTSD after TBI.

At this point, almost all studies looking at the relationship between PTSD and TBI were conducted in adults. Consequently, Mather et al. (2003) explored the relationship between PTSD and presence of mild TBI in children following road traffic accidents. Criteria used by the researchers were children had an age between 6 and 16 years old, currently enrolled in school, and if they had received a mild TBI there was witnessed loss of consciousness and an initial GCS of 13–15 that returned to a full GCS within 24 h of injury. The average age of the 43 participants was 9.7 years, and the sample was comprised of 20 males and 23 females. Twenty of the children were passengers in motor vehicle accidents, 17 were hit as pedestrians, and 6 were on a motorcycle or bicycle. Of the sample, 14 sustained mild TBI and the remaining 29 were classified as not brain injured.

The Children's Posttraumatic Stress Reaction Index (CPTS-RI) was used to measure PTSD symptomatology. The children were also administered the Revised Children's Manifest Anxiety Scale and the Children's Depression Inventory for self-reported anxiety and depression levels, respectively. Parents completed the PTSD module of the Anxiety Disorders Interview Schedule-Children Version to assess their report of their child's PTSD symptomatology, as well as the Child Behavior Checklist (CBCL) to assess internalizing and externalizing behaviors displayed by their children.

Overall, the researchers found that 74 % of children evidenced significant PTSD symptomatology roughly 6 weeks after their accident. There was not a significant difference between those who sustained a mild TBI and those that did not. 86 % of the children with mild TBIs, and 69 % of the children with no brain injury were classified as experiencing significant levels of PTSD symptomatology. This finding is interesting because previous studies with adults suggests that the presence of brain injury decreases the chances of developing PTSD after a traumatic event, however, these results suggest the opposite in children. In regard to comorbidity, children with PTSD were significantly more likely to have higher levels of anxiety and depression.

While the majority of the children had a reduction in PTSD symptomatology over time, one child that initially had no PTSD-like symptoms evidenced severe PTSD at the follow-up assessment. Interestingly, two of this child's siblings that were also involved in the same accident evidenced severe PTSD initially, suggesting that being around their siblings may have caused this child to develop PTSD. Another important factor this study highlights is the accuracy of parental report, which may be detrimental to proper assessment. The researchers found that while 74 % of children endorsed some level of PTSD symptomatology, only 42 % of parents reported significant PTSD symptoms in their children. The authors note that some of this discrepancy may have been due to the difference between the parent report and child report questionnaires, however, it seems that this still only highlights the necessity for careful and thorough evaluations in children.

Military Posttraumatic Stress Disorder and Traumatic Brain Injury. While many researchers still study the relationship between TBI and PTSD, the focus of population has heavily changed. Until the early 2000's most studies were on individuals who received TBIs and PTSD from motor vehicle accidents, assaults, or falling. However, over the past 15 years the focus has changed as a result of the September 11, 2001 terrorists attack on the World Trade Center and the Pentagon. The relationship between PTSD and TBI has become more publicized and discussed now than ever before, with a strong focus on military population. In October, 2001, Operation Enduring Freedom (OEF) was launched, followed by Operation Iraqi Freedom (OIF) in March, 2003. Three additional smaller operations, Operation New Dawn, Operation Inherent Resolve, and Operation Freedom's Sentinel have also been conducted. An estimated 2.7 million military service members have been deployed to war zones since 2001, and more than half of them have been deployed more than once. At least 970,000 veterans have some degree of disability as a result of the wars, and countless live day-to-day with unrecognized physical and psychological scars.

Serving in the military is a dangerous job that presents many opportunities for injury. While in combat areas, soldiers are at constant risk of encountering dangers such as, improvised explosive devices (IEDs), mortar attacks, enemy gunshots, missiles, and physical assaults. With the advancement of protective gear and medical aid, soldiers are surviving injuries that may have proven fatal in the past. Due to the increase of survival from a life threatening experience, there is an increase of soldiers returning with psychological and physiological disorders. For soldiers, open and closed head injuries are a common trepidation that unfortunately becomes a reality for many. Traumatic brain injury (TBI) has commonly been referred to as the signature injury of Operation Enduring Freedom and Operation Iraqi Freedom due to its emerging prevalence. In 2008, approximately one quarter of deployed service members reported head and neck injury, including severe brain trauma (Hoge et al. 2008). Between 10 and 17 % of troops deployed to combat zones have developed PTSD (Sundin et al. 2010). Hoge et al. (2008) found that 43.9 % of soldiers who reported loss of consciousness during battle injury met the requirements for PTSD. With such a high rate of exposure to physically and psychologically traumatic events, exploring the literature on TBI and PTSD in a military population is crucial to understanding these disorders.

Hoge et al. (2008) conducted one of the most prominent studies on mild TBI in returning U.S. soldiers to date. The focus of their study was on the prevalence and significance of self-reported history of combat-related mild TBI among soldiers after a year long deployment to Iraq. They sought to provide information that would further the literature on prevention and treatment strategies. In-depth questionnaires were sent to 4618 U.S. Army soldiers, from which 2525 soldiers were ultimately included in the study. The questionnaire asked whether or not the soldiers had been injured during deployment, what they were injured by, whether they received a mild TBI from the accident, and immediate symptoms of their accident (loss of consciousness, seeing stars, confusion, etc.). Combat intensity was measured using 17 of the 18 questions from the Combat Experiences Scale. Soldiers were asked to rate their overall health, and also completed the Patient Health Questionnaire 15-item somatic symptom severity scale (PHQ-15). An additional five questions were asked regarding post-concussive symptoms about memory, balance, concentration, ringing in the ears, and irritability. Depression and PTSD were assessed by using the 9-item depression assessment module of the PHQ and the 17-item National Center for PTSD Checklist, respectively.

Overall, 4.9 % of soldiers reported an injury with loss of consciousness, while 10.3 % endorsed an injury with an altered mental status without loss of consciousness. Hoge et al. (2008) found that soldiers who endorsed mild TBI were significantly more likely to report a blast mechanism of injury, exposure to more than one explosion, high combat intensity, and hospitalization. As already noted, 43.9 % of soldiers who reported loss of consciousness during battle injury met the requirements for PTSD. 27 % of those with an altered mental status but no loss of consciousness met criteria for PTSD. It was found that loss of consciousness and combat intensity were the only two factors significantly associated with PTSD symptomatology. Consistent with literature from civilian population, injury with loss of consciousness was significantly related to the development of major depressive disorder, as well as poorer general health. So overall, soldiers with mild TBI reported significantly higher rates of physical and mental health problems, and injuries with loss of consciousness resulted in a much greater risk of health problems.

Although numerous studies show that PTSD and TBI have a high comorbidity rate, very few truly take a look at the accuracy and best method of assessment for these disorders. There is currently no definitive method for determining which symptoms are due TBI and which are due to PTSD. While some symptoms are more clear-cut than others, there are numerous common symptoms that could go either way. It has been suggested that one method of segregating PTSD from TBI symptoms would be conducting PTSD or TBI specific treatment to see which symptoms subside and which remain. Although initially this seems like a possible solution, various researchers argue that due to the "biological interface" that suggests a physiological correlation between PTSD and TBI, treatment may alleviate both TBI and PTSD symptoms, in turn, providing inconclusive results (Church and Palmer-Hoffman 2014; Kennedy et al. 2007).

On the other hand, Church and Palmer-Hoffman (2014) raise the point that the results of such treatment may in actually just highlight the difficulties we have in distinguishing between such disorders and the lack of knowledge we have in the treatment capabilities for TBI and PTSD individually. Church and Palmer-Hoffman (2014) sought to examine whether etiology (PTSD or TBI) was important in terms of treatment outcomes by providing emotional freedom techniques (EFT) coaching to 59 veterans with PTSD, to determine whether the resolution of PTSD symptoms would correlate with a reduction in TBI symptoms. Emotional freedom technique is a brief exposure therapy with somatic and cognitive components. During this treatment method, patients are asked to pair the memory of a traumatic event with a statement of self-acceptance, while simultaneously stimulating 12 different acupressure points with finger tips. The researchers noted that while EFT has been shown to meet APA's Division 12 criteria for empirically supported treatments as a "well-established treatment" for PTSD, little is known of the impact it may have on TBI symptomatology.

Of the 59 veterans, 30 comprised the EFT group while 29 made up the wait-list control group. Participants completed assessments at baseline, after three sessions, after six sessions, and at 3- and 6-month follow-ups. Posttraumatic stress disorder symptoms were screened for by using the global severity index and positive symptom total on the Symptom Assessment-45, while the PCL-M (PTSD Checklist-Military version) was used at each assessment. The authors indicated that because there is no generally accepted brief TBI screener, nine items from the Patient Health Questionnaire somatoform module of the Primary Care Evaluation of Mental Disorders (PRIME-MD), along with a list of 17 TBI symptoms were used to assess for TBI. After isolating TBI and somatoform symptoms, analyses indicated a significant reduction in TBI symptoms after three EFT sessions, and further reductions were shown after six sessions. The reductions in symptoms were maintained after 3-months and 6-months. Many individuals who have sustained a mild TBI still report experiencing postconcussive symptoms (headache, fatigue, memory difficulties) years after their injury. However, in Church and Palmer-Hoffman's (2014) sample, both somatoform symptoms and TBI symptoms were significantly reduced. While there are certainly limitations to their study, the results still shed light on just how little we still know about the relationship between TBI and PTSD, as well as our ability to differentiate etiology of symptomatology.

Screeners and questionnaires are often used in medical and private practice settings due to their time efficiency and low cost, allowing clinicians to quickly and relatively cheaply gain insight into a client on multiple domains. While presenting and brief history of symptoms are crucial to an evaluation, these components are only pieces to the puzzle. In addition to understanding all of the present symptoms, a clinician must take a detailed history of the client and their traumatic event. Lange et al. (2014) sought to identify factors that are predictive of the endorsement of PTSD and postconcussive symptoms after a TBI in a military population. The researchers looked at a total of 22 factors related to demographic variables, injury circumstances, injury severity, treatment/evaluation, and psychological/physical symptoms.

Participants of the study were 1600 U.S. service members who sustained a mild to moderate TBI and were evaluated by the Defense and Veterans Brain Injury Center. Diagnosis and classification of TBI severity was primarily conducted by a

Physician's Assistant or Nurse who were trained to evaluate the presence and severity of TBI. The medical professionals determined severity and presence by conducting a comprehensive clinical screening that consisted of a patient interview, a comprehensive medical chart review, case conferencing, and a family interview and collection of other collateral information. Loss of consciousness (LOC), post-traumatic amnesia (PTA), and alteration of consciousness (AOC) were used to classify TBI severity. The authors reported that GCS scores were not available.

For a classification of moderate TBI one must have had a LOC for longer than 30 min to 24 h, PTA for 1–7 days, and the presence or absence of intracranial abnormality. Complicated mild TBI was classified as a LOC for less than or equal to 30 min, PTA for less than 24 h, and the presence of intracranial abnormality. Uncomplicated mild TBI had the same criteria, except for the need of an absence of intracranial abnormality. Equivocal mild TBI was classified by having no PTA or LOC, with a present AOC. Additionally, the Neurobehavioral Symptom Inventory (NSI), a 22-item measure that evaluates self-reported postconcussive symptoms, was utilized for assessing the presence and severity of TBI. The PCL-C Version, a 17-item self-report measure, was used for evaluating PTSD symptoms.

Overall, the authors found four factors to be statistically related to postconcussive symptom endorsement. The four factors were as follows: low bodily injury severity, posttraumatic stress symptoms, depression, and being wounded during a military operation related to the Global War on Terrorism (GWOT), with depression and posttraumatic stress symptoms as the most strongly associated with clinical elevations in postconcussive symptoms accounting for 41.5 % of the variance. Interestingly, brain injury severity was not associated with symptom reporting following TBI.

This study supports the findings of other studies that suggest PTSD and depression largely explain the relation between a history of TBI and postconcussion symptoms reporting. Lange et al. (2013) that clinically meaningful postconcussion symptom reporting occurs only 5.6 % of the time when there is an absence of these four factors: (1) symptom exaggeration, (2) poor cognitive effort, (3) depression, and (4) traumatic stress. If anything, the work of Lange and colleagues shed light on the numerous factors that must be taken into consideration when evaluating individuals that present with TBI.

As discussed earlier in this chapter, understanding the ramifications of being exposed to blasts are still in its infancy stages. Lippa et al. (2010) conducted profile analyses to explore the differences in self-reported postconcussive symptoms in 339 veterans reporting mild TBI dependent upon their mechanism of injury (blast only, nonblast only, or both blast and nonblast), distance from the blast, and number of blast injuries. The criteria used for mild TBI in this study were a self-reported LOC of 30 min or less, or disorientation for 24 h or less, following a credible injury mechanism. The NSI was used to measure postconcussive symptoms, and symptoms of PTSD were measured using the National Center for PTSD 17-item checklist (PCL). The PCL was developed to correspond with the Diagnostic and Statistical Manual-Fourth Edition (DSM-IV 1994). Similarly to Lange et al. (2014), the authors found that PTSD symptoms accounted for a considerable portion of variance in postconcussive symptom report. Additionally, it was discovered that PTSD is more common in those with histories of blast-related TBIs than those with nonblast-related TBIs. However, neither the number of blast injuries nor the distance from the blast was correlated to total PTSD symptoms reported.

Neuroanatomy of PTSD with TBI

The advancement of technology has allowed researchers to explore the brain in a whole new way. Some studies have used functional magnetic resonance imaging (fMRI) and found that individuals with PTSD and mild TBI share abnormalities in the frontal lobes, more specifically the dorsolateral prefrontal, orbitofrontal, medial frontal, and the anterior cingulate cortex (Shu et al. 2014; Simmons and Matthews 2011; Stein and McAllister 2009). Individually, patients with PTSD tend to have hyperactivity in the medial frontal and anterior cingulate areas (Carrion et al. 2008; Matthews et al. 2011; Swick et al. 2012), while the neuroanatomical differences in those with mild TBI only vary case by case. Shu et al. (2014) utilized electroencephalography (EEG) to test whether those with PTSD and TBI share abnormal activation in various frontal regions, specifically the anterior cingulate cortex.

The researchers believe that PTSD symptomatology may particularly mediated by the anterior cingulate cortex, and this difference may be apparent during cognitive control tasks that require response inhibition. Participants were composed of 32 combat veterans, 17 with a mild TBI and PTSD, 15 with a mild TBI and no PTSD. A stop task was performed by each participant during EEG monitoring, requiring the inhibition of initiated motor responses. Interestingly, Shu et al. (2014) found that those with PTSD and mild TBI had a greater inhibitory processing event related potential (ERP) in the dorsal anterior cingulate. The researchers concluded that in veterans with mild TBI, larger ERPs in the dorsal anterior cingulate are associated with higher PTSD symptom endorsement. They continued to explain that this relationship is likely related to complications with controlling ongoing brain processes, including thoughts and consequently feelings about their trauma.

Yeh et al. (2014) investigated the differences in white matter between blast and impact injury, along with the impact of postconcussion and PTSD symptoms. Participants were 37 US service members, comprising of 29 with mild, 7 with moderate, and 1 with severe TBI; 17 experienced blast trauma and 20 were considered nonblast. TBI evaluations included a patient interview, a comprehensive medical chart review, case conferencing, and a family interview for collateral information. The diagnosis of TBI was based on the presence of duration of LOC, PTA, AOC, and neuroimaging. Mild TBI was considered as AOC or LOC for 30 min or less, or PTA for less than 24 h and no radiological abnormalities. Moderate TBI criteria were comprised of positive neuroimaging findings, PTA for more than 24 h, or LOC for more than 30 min. Finally, severe TBI was diagnosed for those with PTA for longer than one week or LOC for more than 1 day. Postconcussion was assessed for by using the

NSI, and the PCL-C was used for PTSD. Diffusion tensor imaging (DTI) was used to assess the neurocircuitry by fiber tracking and tract-specific analysis, along with region of interest analysis. Overall, for both blast and nonblast patients, the most common white matter injury was in the fronto-striatal and fronto-limbic circuits, along with the fronto-parieto-occipital association fibers.

The researchers reported finding significant differences between the blast and nonblast groups in subcortical tracks. Specifically, subcortical superior–inferiorly oriented tracks were more susceptible to blast injury, while anterior-posteriorly oriented tracks were more impacted by direct force trauma. In regards to the influence of PTSD and subconcussive symptoms, the tractography revealed higher endorsement of both PTSD and subconcussive symptoms was associated with low fractional anisotropy in the major nodes of compromised cortico-striatal-thalamic-cerebellar-cortical (CSTCC) network.

TBI, PTSD, and Alzheimer's Disease

Numerous studies have linked TBI to an increased chance of developing Alzheimer's disease, as well as causing an earlier onset for Alzheimer's disease (Bilbul and Schipper 2011; Jellinger 2004; Johnson et al. 2010; Lye and Shores 2000). Likewise, some studies have found a correlation between presence of PTSD and development of dementia (Qureshi et al. 2010; Yaffe et al. 2010). Yaffe et al. (2010) found that those diagnosed as having PTSD were at almost double the risk of developing dementia compared with those without PTSD. They posed that PTSD might be involved in accelerating the aging of the brain, being that PTSD often last late into life and has been found to cause hypothalamic–pituitary–adrenal axis dysfunction. These researchers also discussed how some have found that veterans with PTSD have smaller hippocampal volumes, which have been shown to correlate with deficits in short-term memory performance. Since smaller hippocampal volumes are associated with poor cognitive function and increased risk of dementia in healthy elderly people, it may be argued that PTSD causes hippocampal atrophy, which in turn increases risk of cognitive decline and dementia. Yaffe et al. (2010) also points out that it is also possible a smaller hippocampus is a predisposition factor for both PTSD and dementia.

Weiner et al. (2014) are currently conducting a investigating the relationship between PTSD, TBI, and Alzheimer's disease. Since both PTSD and TBI have been independently associated with Alzheimer's disease, the present researchers hypothesize that TBI and/or PTSD reduce cognitive reserve, causing greater cognitive impairment after adjusting for age, education, prewar cognitive functioning, brain amyloid load, and hippocampal volume; and that there will be significant relationships between severity of PTSD and TBI and greater cognitive impairment. All participants will be administered the Clinician Administered PTSD Scale (CAPS) to identify PTSD symptomatology, along with a full battery of neuropsychological tests comprised of the Montreal Cognitive Assessment, everyday cognition, the

Mini-Mental State Examination, the Alzheimer's Disease Assessment Scale-Cognitive 13, the Logical Memory Test I and II, the Boston Naming Test, the Category Fluency Test, the Clock Drawing Test, the American National Adult Reading Test, the Auditory Verbal Learning Test, the Trail Making Test Parts A and B, the Clinical Dementia Rating, the Activities of Daily Living/Functional Assessment Questionnaire, the Neuropsychiatric Inventory, and the Geriatric Depression Scale. Additionally, cerebrospinal fluid (CSF) will be obtained at baseline using a lumbar puncture. Both amyloid PET images and MRI will be performed. Currently, participants are still being recruited; however, to date, this appears to be the largest study to look in-depth at the neurological and neuropsychological relationship between PTSD, TBI, and Alzheimer's disease.

Chapter 3
Designing a Neuropsychological Battery

Selecting a battery. There is no single test battery that is used by everyone or even a majority of people working on these issues. Neuropsychology offers a wide range of tests across many areas which can be considered by users. Tests selected from each area if any depends on the training and preferences of each user and the specific population being studied.

For the PTSD-TBI comparison, however, there appear some areas which are essential to the understanding of the client. In many settings, this comprehensive approach may be short circuited based on issues of time and availability of personnel. For example, in military settings where large number of screenings may be required, it may seem impossible to do full battery testing in a timely manner. As can be seen in the research cites in Chap. 2, this may reduce evaluations to short questionnaires which rely on the truthfulness and insight of the individual being studied. In the populations being studied here, individuals may be unaware consciously of their own problems and/or may choose to blame everything on one factor (more often TBI than emotional factors). In the cognitive realm, computerized screening tests may be used which are better developed to detect acute TBI factors in individuals, who are highly motivated to do well than with an injury than with the long-term cognitive sequelae of TBI in a population whose motivation and effort may be more variable. Although such tests are indeed useful for specific purposes, they can never be seen as measuring the same things as more complex tests as those which will be discussed here.

Another related issue is effort and motivation. While such tests are almost universally required in clinical settings, they are rarely used in research based on the apparent belief that no one would fake good or bad or that these effects would be random in the final outcome. In an individual clinical assessment, such factors can seriously distort the outcome of an examination. In the case of accident victims, there is often

© The Author(s) 2016
C.J. Golden et al., *The Intercorrelation of Traumatic Brain Injury and PTSD in Neuropsychological Evaluations*, SpringerBriefs in Behavioral Criminology, DOI 10.1007/978-3-319-47033-7_3

a forensic process involved, ranging from collecting from an insurance company to a substantial, adversarial lawsuit, or simply anger at those involved in the accident. In addition, effort can be impacted by pain, loss of sleep, depression, and irritability which can arise because of non-brain related-physical symptoms. Each of these can substantially change test results if not clearly considered.

In military individuals, we also see several factors affecting effort and cooperation. While forensics are less, the individual may be motivated by the likelihood of a service connected disability or the role a disorder may have on the possibility of promotion. Unique to the military assessments is a client wanting to deny impact of a disorder so they can return to their unit. Soldiers have told me that not returning to their unit is abandoning their comrades, especially in a combat area. On the other hand, some soldiers are so adversely affected by their experiences they do not wish to return under any conditions, whether or not they meet criteria for TBI or PTSD. As with other clients, issues like fatigue or lack of sleep may impact results.

Areas for Evaluation

Intelligence. An intellectual evaluation is required in all evaluations. Over the years, there have been very different conceptualizations of what intelligence is. In a number of these conceptualizations, IQ is looked upon as a biological limit on what a person is able to achieve. In the context of testing, IQ is perhaps best viewed as a person's average ability across a wide range of cognitive tasks. In this view, cognitive skills are not seen as all the same but rather a range of strengths and weaknesses which are largely normally distributed so that half the skills are stronger and half are weaker. Two-thirds of all scores should be within one standard deviation of the IQ score (15 points if we use the standard intelligence testing scoring system), while one-sixths should be strengths above this range and one-sixths should be weaknesses below this range. This gives a good starting point to evaluate whether there have been actual changes in the pattern of cognitive skills.

Ideally, this should be measured by one of the standardized intellectual test batteries as this gives us a better estimate of what the true IQ level may be. While individualized tests of vocabulary or matrix reasoning are used to estimate premorbid IQ (as these tests are thought to be less impaired by TBI) they do not give a comprehensive view of the range of cognitive skills. They may be used to estimate premorbid IQ, as can such factors as educational level, standardized achievement tests from high school or college, and standardized intelligence tests taken by the military during the enlistment process. Intelligence tests are thought to primarily measure cognitive functions which represent the posterior areas of the brain (although this is an oversimplification).

Memory. Memory is a necessary area but difficult to assess reliability in individuals with these diagnoses. Most memory tests also require attention and concentration and effort over time more so than other tests. Many tests also are affected by the strategies which the person uses, with some strategies causing inefficient results but do not reflect memory but rather organizational and planning skills. While memory is a basic function of subcortical areas such as the hippocampus, the approach to the memory task is dominated by cortical areas. They are also likely to cause more anxiety and bring up expectations of failure as most clients with TBI/PTSD expect to do poorly on memory tests even if their own memory problems are primarily around their injury or are vague in nature. Such expectations of failure need to be considered in selecting tests as there are several frequently used tests which are quite demanding of time and effort and give the impression of being very difficult. Both verbal and nonverbal memory should be sampled, as should delayed and immediate memory.

Executive skills. Executive skills are often impaired after TBI and are seen as impaired in cases of PTSD as well. Because executive skills are really a large conglomeration of individual skills not all of which are sampled by any single tests, a range of tests must be used to sample the major skills. These include skills as diverse as focused and sustained attention, inhibition, emotional control, emotional stability, the ability to distinguish reality from fantasy, insight, flexibility, planning, performance evaluation, complex problem solving, organization, and other similar higher level skills which go beyond those skills tested in intellectual tests (biological intelligence rather than psychometric intelligence in the words of Ward Halstead). These skills are mediated by the frontal lobes and their connections to the subcortical areas of the brain and the anterior temporal lobe in a complex interplay of basic subcortical structures sending neuronal impulses upward to the frontal lobes and dampening and modifying signals flowing downward from the cognitive areas of the frontal lobe.

While cognitive structures are located in the cortical areas, their functions are interfered with or aided by signals stretching upward from the subcortical structures. These areas are easily disrupted by TBI due to the large number of neuronal interactions required for even basic skills which require a precise timing of neuronal interactions easily disrupted by blast and acceleration type injuries and whose recovery is complex and often poorly addressed by rehabilitation which focuses on more immediate deficits in self-care and memory. As noted, no single test measures all of these functions, so a range of tests is necessary to sample as many as possible, but not in a manner which over stresses the client, a delicate balance in which tests without time limits are preferred when possible.

Personality tests. It is clear that one wishes to measure a personality or emotional disorder, measures of emotional, and personality function must be included. Traditionally dating back to the Halstead–Reitan, the MMPI was included although in practice was often subservient to the cognitive tests in reaching diagnoses and other conclusions. Despite attempts to find ways to do so, the MMPI has not been successful in identifying item or scale patterns which define whether a disorder is neurological or emotional. Much of this research was based on the assumption that all cases were either one or the other, ignoring the possibility that both conditions could be present. Thus, while the tests may present information about emotional functioning, they rarely yield information on etiology.

While objective tests have been preferred, for their ease in scoring and administration, as well as the ease in doing research, the MMPI and similar tests have significant limitations, as the results are often based on the insight and intentions of the test takers. While validity scales are included in the MMPI and many other tests which have been used (e.g. the MCMI or PAI) more intelligent individuals can respond in invalid ways without being clearly identified. Other tests (like the Beck Depression Inventory) do not contain any validity scales and can be easily manipulated. Clients may respond truthfully to these tests but that perception is based on their perception of what is wrong with them: a TBI client may blame their problems on PTSD, and thus exaggerate those symptoms they think are associated with PTSD and minimize the symptoms they think are associated with TBI. Contrarily, another client will minimize PTSD symptoms while exaggerating TBI symptoms. These clients are not malingering, but rather conforming their symptoms to their expectations. In the days of the Internet—when any individual can look up the symptoms of TBI, PTSD, or any other disorder—such a confirmatory bias towards a disorder can easily be supported without the intention to deceive. Nevertheless the results, while looking valid, are misleading.

To deal with this, some have become advocates of tests like the PAI or MCMI, tests which are more face-valid than the MMPI and therefore more easily manipulated (but also shorter to save time in the examination). As noted above, shorter more face-valid questionnaires as used in the research cited in Chap. 2 are also questionable because they are even more easily manipulated and include no validity scales. The remaining alternative is projective tests, a controversial choice as many psychologists object to tests which are not objective. Projective tests are harder to give properly and immensely more difficult to score properly and to research, yet they remain common among those who specialize in personality assessment. The major reason for this is that they are not easily manipulated although clients can refuse to give honest answers) and that the client may reveal emotional issues which they consciously deny or repress.

Achievement Test. While some sort of achievement test is frequently found in many test batteries, they may not be appropriate or needed in the kinds of cases discussed here. Educational functions are rarely disrupted directly by either TBI or PTSD, although clients may appear to do poorly because of attentional or anxiety-related problems. This, however, rarely adds anything useful to the diagnostic workup. Word recognition tests can be used to estimate premorbid IQ but that can also be done with Vocabulary or Matrix tests included in common intellectual test batteries.

Tests of effort. While a test like the MMPI includes its own validity scales, these scales are not effective in predicting effort on cognitive tests or in detecting the consistent but insightless client who may be seen in this population. Thus, a test of effort which is aimed at cognitive tests is necessary, one which looks sufficiently complex but is in fact quite easy. Some effort tests are quite easy and look easy, so such tests should be avoided. The ideal test is one which appears difficult, but in fact can be completed by most people, even those with head injuries and at lower levels of intelligence. In addition, there are a variety of stand-alone tests aimed at assessing motivation or deception in emotional evaluation, one of which is recommended to be included in the evaluation of these clients.

Motor and sensory skills. Although motor and sensory skill tests are often included in neuropsychological test battery, they make most sense in cases of stroke or other highly localized lesions where clearly lateralized lesions are present. Such deficits are much rarer in accident cases except where there is direct damage to a localized area through shrapnel, a bullet, or focal bleeding within the brain tissue. In all of these cases, the presence of a brain injury is rarely debated, so the issue is not diagnosis of a brain injury but rather an assessment of the cognitive and emotional aspects of the injury. These tests rarely give valuable data although more complex tests may give insight to the interactions of cognitive and motor behavior.

Administration Issues

Before turning to our specific test recommendations, there are some general principles necessary in working with these populations in order to get accurate test results. It must be remembered that administration "rules" in test manuals are set for the normal population, with the assumption that everyone is motivated to do their best and can follow the test rules without frequent repetition. Their procedures also assume that individuals are at their best: well rested, alert, cooperative, and motivated. When these assumptions are not true, clients fail to do their best and the data becomes misleading. When our goal is to make an accurate diagnosis, we cannot nor should we follow directions slavishly simply for the sake of following them. Changes must be made designed to get a client's best performance so we can understand the underlying factors to their disorder.

This does not mean we can run roughshod over standardized directions or scoring as they are designed to allow us to compare performance to others. Some things can easily be ignored—if a test provides for only one repetition of the instructions at the beginning, it will generally not affect the testing to repeat the instructions to the client who forgets what to do due to memory or anxiety or distractibility issues. On the other hand, in a memory test, repeating the memory items when not allowed will introduce additional phantom trials which will change the results. However, before administering each trial, one can make sure that the client is paying attention and ready for the trial.

With this in mind, there are several rules one can follow to insure maximum, accurate, and valid performance which aids in the most precise diagnosis. These rules include: (1) Always make sure the client understands the direction. In most cases, one can paraphrase directions, but without providing additional information. Repeat directions as necessary if the client becomes confused or forgets; (2) While scoring should always be done based on time limits, if the client is slow but appears to be working and accurate, allow the client more time, but noting their performance when the time limit is up. This can give the client a sense of accomplishment if they are negative about their performance. However, if the client is frustrated by an item or clearly doing poorly, it is best not to let the item continue as it may affect future tests; (3) In a few cases, an item can be ended early if the client is very frustrated and clearly doing poorly, such as on the more complex items of Block Design or Similarities; (4) Praise the clients performance liberally, whether the answer is correct or not except in those cases where the correct answer is obvious to the client; (5) Some tests, like the Wechsler Intelligence Scales, have suggested starting points at slightly more difficult items. For clients who are easily frustrated or upset, start with the first and easiest items to allow the client to have more success and feel more comfortable; (6) In timed tests where the client clearly does not know what to do or fails to follow instructions, stop the test quickly, and give another time; (7) If the client is impaired by lack of sleep (common in both PTSD and trauma pain cases), do not administer timed tests or tests requiring substantial concentration until the client is better rested or composed. Test results from an exhausted client are meaningless diagnostically; (8) When a client becomes excessively anxious, angry, or frustrated, discontinue testing an appropriate place (not in the middle of a speeded item) and calm the client down before continuing. If the client cannot be calmed down, discontinue testing until a better time; (9) In preparing clients for speeded tests, make sure they understand the importance of going as fast as possible prior to starting the test or item; (10) Make sure clients understand that they will miss items, because tests are designed to see how much difficulty is required to make one miss items so that everyone misses items; (11) Be on the alert for sudden breaks in attention which could suggest the presence of seizures interfering with consciousness. Try to reorient a client in such situations through verbal or gestural cues to see if they respond. Low level, brief seizures are often missed because they can be so fleeting; (12) Never say anything negative about a client's performance, but you can ask if they are feeling able to continue testing; (13) Encourage guessing on all tests, noting that we never penalize for guessing. Clients will stop prematurely on items such as memory tests because they are afraid of making errors. Encourage and praise clients for guessing whether the guesses are right or wrong; (14) On tests with time limits, prompt for answer before the time runs out; (15) Actively interact with clients rather than just mechanically give tests so that they are engaged—it is recognized in therapy that a good relationship with clients aids therapeutic outcome. This is often true in testing as well; (16) When clients make errors, keep abreast as much of you can of the type of error made. While such information is not required by most tests, it can offer useful insights into the underlying mechanism of the errors. For example, if digit symbol coding is performed slowly, it is because the client is compulsive about doing, careful accurate renderings or are they meteorically unable to produce the right shapes or do they become confused about what they are doing or something else entirely? Similarly, when they get a right answer in an odd way, note how they achieve the answer. For example, get the arithmetic item correct by counting on their fingers.

Using these techniques effectively will increase the usefulness of the cognitive data, yielding a better picture of what a client can do (which may be limited by brain damage) versus what a client does (limited by many emotional and motivational elements). In most of these cases, effective use of the techniques requires more training as well as more flexibility. While a CT scan can be done regardless of the patient's mood or feelings (if they will lay still!) and so can be scheduled inflexibly, neuropsychological, and psychological testing depends upon the cooperation, motivation, and involvement of the client. Therefore inflexibility, while good for running an institution or private practice, is not amenable to producing credible results. In addition, while screening tests have uses when large numbers of people must be screened for a specific purpose, they are not appropriate for finer distinctions as called for here. Similarly, current computer batteries taken by the client alone without detailed observation are not a substitute for a combination of appropriately administered one-on-one tests with trained observation and integration.

Finally, when these techniques are used other than incidentally they need to be listed in the Behavioral Observations/Test Observations section of a report. They are valuable so the reader can both understand what was done as well as understand what is required to get maximal performance out of an individual. This information can be very helpful in planning intervention techniques and approaches with the client in any rehabilitation setting.

Selecting the Test Battery

As noted previously, there is not only one test battery which can fit these criteria. No test battery can measure everything in every way without taking forever and must be adapted to the client. This battery assumes client whose premorbid functioning was in the 70+ IQ range and could function at least marginally. Those beginning at a lower level or severely injured would benefit from an alternate battery s would individuals with pronounced aphasia or severe upper motor problems. The following tests and summaries represent the main battery we employ in this population, augmented (or shortened) as necessitated by a given case.

Wechsler Adult Intelligence Scale—Fourth Edition (WAIS-IV)

The Wechsler Adult Intelligence Scale—Fourth Edition is a measure of general intellectual functioning and consists of 15 subtests, 5 of which are optional. The Verbal Comprehension Index measures verbal conceptualization, knowledge, and expression along with the measures and the ability to analyze information and solve problems using language-based reasoning. Similarities requires the examinee to identify how two objects or concepts are similar/alike/what they have in common and measures verbal conceptualization ability, and abstract verbal skills/reasoning. Vocabulary requires the examinee to define the vocabulary words of increasing difficulties and measures verbal conceptualization ability, acquired knowledge, and verbal concept formation. Information requires the examinee to answer questions about general factual information; answer questions on a broad range of general knowledge topics. This measures their ability to acquire, retain, and retrieve general factual knowledge.

The Perceptual Organization/Reasoning Index measures nonverbal thinking and motor coordination, using visual-spatial and visual-motor skills to solve nonschool taught problems and the ability to solve novel problems that do not depend on formal schooling. Block Design requires the examinee to replicate pictures using blocks and assesses the ability to perceive and analyze designs by breaking the whole into parts and utilizes visual-constructive skills, nonverbal reasoning, and spatial ability/perception. Matrix Reasoning requires the examinee to look at a matrix and identify the missing piece from among five choices. It measures spatial ability, visual-spatial pattern analysis and the ability to utilize nonverbal abstract problem solving and inductive reasoning. Visual Puzzles requires the examinee to look at a completed puzzle and select three responses that reconstruct the puzzle. Hypothetically, this new subtest measures visual-spatial organization, construction, attention to detail, nonverbal reasoning, spatial ability.

Working Memory Index is a measure of attention and ability to manipulate orally presented sequences, to temporarily retain information in memory, to perform some operation or manipulation with it, and to produce a result. Digit Span requires the examinee to repeat sequences of orally presented numbers and has three components. The forward portion involves rote learning and memory, attention, encoding, and auditory processing. The backward portion involves working memory, transformation of information, mental manipulation, and visuospatial imaging. The sequencing portion involves working memory, transformation of information, and visuospatial imaging. Arithmetic requires an examinee to mentally calculate answers to simple arithmetic word problems under timed conditions. This measures mental manipulation, concentration, attention, mental alertness, short and long-term memory, and numerical reasoning ability.

The Processing Speed Index measures speed, sustained attention, memory, speed of thinking, and motor speed. Symbol Search requires the examinee to need to scan a series of shapes and identify whether any of the shapes match. This measures processing speed, short-term visual memory, visual-motor coordination, and visual discrimination. Digit Symbol Coding requires the examinee to match numbers with symbols using a provided key under timed conditions. The subtest measures speed, memory, and sustained attention.

Wechsler Memory Scale—Fourth Edition (WMS-IV)

The Wechsler Memory Scale—Fourth Edition is a test of an individual's visual, verbal, and working memory functioning in persons ages 16–90. The WMS-IV is designed to measure aspects of memory that are commonly seen in those with memory deficits or neurological, developmental, and psychiatric disorders. The WMS-IV is composed of seven subtests, with four of the subtests utilizing an immediate and delayed aspect. The Brief Cognitive Status Exam is an optional subtest wherein the examinee performs tasks to aid in measuring recall, inhibitory control, clock drawing, orientation to time, and verbal fluency. Within the Logical Memory subtest two short stories are presented orally and after each story the examinee is asked to recall as much of the story as they can remember, assessing for immediate narrative memory. The delayed portion is given 20–30 min later, asking the examinee to recall as much of the stories as they can remember and assesses long-term narrative memory. A recognition subtest requires them to answer yes/no to questions about the stories. Verbal-paired Associates requires the examinee to recall 14 word pairs to assess for immediate verbal memory, 4 trials consisting of the same word pairs in a different order are administered. The delayed portion assesses long-term verbal information in both a cued and recognition manner. For the Designs subtest, the examinee is shown a grid with 4–8 designs, the grid is removed and the y are asked to select the designs from a set of cards (that included distractors) and place them in the same position on the grid as they previously saw. This subtest is intended to measure spatial memory for novel information. The delayed portion assesses visual memory and long-term spatial memory and includes a free recall and a recognition task. Visual Reproduction measures memory for nonverbal visual stimuli. The examinee is shown five designs, one at a time, for 10 s each and is asked to immediately draw the design from memory. The delayed portion, given 20–30 later requires them to draw the designs, from free recall and also includes a recognition section. The Spatial Addition subtest assess visual-spatial working memory as the examinee is shown two grids, back to back, with blue and red circles and is required to add or subtract the location of the circles. The Symbol Span subtest assesses visual working memory for novel visual stimuli. Overall Index scores for Auditory Memory, Visual Memory, Visual Working Memory, Immediate Memory, and Delayed Memory are provided.

Memory scores lower than 80 would suggest difficulty with activities of daily living such as cooking, driving, and handling finances. It is recommended that a person obtain supervision and use memory lists. Memory scores lower than 70 suggest incompetence to manage own affairs, supervision for all activities of daily living, no driving or management of finances, and appointment of a legal guardian. When memory is greater than intellectual abilities, that signifies a functional psychiatric disorder whereas intellectual abilities greater than memory abilities signifies a CNS disease affecting memory (Mittenberg 2015).

Structured Interview of Reported Symptoms—Second Edition (SIRS-2)

The Structured Interview of Reported Symptoms—Second Edition (SIRS-2) is a measure utilized for the assessment of feigned mental disorders within the older adolescent and adult populations. The test was normed on individuals with normal or borderline intellectual functioning; however, the manual states that those with mild intellectual disabilities have successfully taken the measure. The developers suggest knowledge of the individual's verbal abilities in determining their potential for relevant responses. The SIRS-2 uses eight primary scales in order to discriminate feigning. The eight scales each measure different aspects such as endorsement of symptoms that do not occur often, endorsing a combination of symptoms not typically found together, endorsing preposterous symptoms, endorsing symptoms as a major issue, reporting common psychological problems as major issues, not being selective with symptom reporting, deeming symptoms as unbearable, reporting more pathology than observed. The manual clearly states that "genuine and feigned mental disorders are not mutually exclusive categories. The mere presence of feigning does not preclude the presence of a severe mental disorder" (Rogers et al. 2010, p. 31). Feigning is classified as gross exaggeration or fabrication of psychopathology while genuine responding is an appropriate effort to describe symptoms and psychopathology without exaggeration. For example, an individual could have a true diagnosis of PTSD, but have a secondary gain, such as disability income, that would lead them to feign. The SIRS-2 is based on the opinion that false positives is a much more egregious error than false negatives and have adjusted their cutoff scores to minimize false positive errors.

Category Test

The Category Test is a computerized evaluative tool used to measure nonverbal concept formation and the ability to shift and maintain problem-solving strategies. The Category Test consists of seven subtests, each with a series of stimuli that suggests a number from 1 to 4. The difficulty of the task changes throughout each subtest and the examinee is required to guess the strategy necessary to solve the problem in order to obtain the correct answer. The examinee is given only one chance for each stimulus and the only feedback that is provided is the computer generating the sound of a bell for correct and a buzzer for incorrect responses. Using this feedback, the examinee must alter his analysis until he is able to continuously provide the correct answer.

Test of Memory Malingering (TOMM)

The Test of Memory Malingering is used to assess the degree of effort displayed by a client on memory tasks. The TOMM purports to assists clinicians in discriminating between genuine memory impairments and malingerers. The test has two learning trials, each consisting of 50 drawings (presented for 3 s each, 1 picture at a time) and 50 recognition pages. On the recognition pages, two pictures are shown, one previously presented picture and a new picture, requiring the individual to choose the correct target picture. There is a third trial, retention, which only consists of recognition pages with no administration of the target pictures. Typically, the two learning trials are adequate to assess malingering, but the retention trial is utilized to validate the results. The TOMM is insensitive to neurological impairments while remaining sensitive to malingering with research on head injured individuals and those with intellectual disabilities scoring above the recommended cutoff score. A concern with interpretation of the TOMM is that some clinicians believe a low score automatically means malingering when in reality it could be due to low motivation or effort. Administration error can also produce low results if a clinician is not making sure the individual is actually focused on the stimuli. Some clinicians see this as a measure that does not take a lot of effort on behalf of the individual, but this is not true and the test should not be administered when an individual is fatigued as the results may prove invalid. It is important to remember that malingering demonstrates intentional exaggeration or falsification and the TOMM alone should not be the only instrument utilized in the determination.

Millon Clinical Multiaxial Inventory-III (MCMI-III)

The Millon Clinical Multiaxial Inventory-III is a self-report measure that assesses a wide range of information related to personality, emotional adjustment, and attitude toward taking tests. The MCMI-III personality scales are based on Millon's theory of personality and Axis I disorders are based on the framework of his theories. The MCMI-III groups the scales into personality and psychopathology categories between Axis I and Axis II. While the DSM-5 no longer utilizes the 5 axis system, this classification is still useful in determining whether a person is suffering from a personality disorder or an acute clinical disorder. The personality scales are also further grouped with the intention of separating out severity of psychopathology. Consequently, Schizotypal, Borderline, and personality scales are separated from the 11 basic personality scales and moderately severe Clinical Syndromes are separated from Thought Disorder, Major Depression, and Delusional Disorder, which are considered the more Severe Clinical Syndromes and may constitute a psychotic thought process. Given that scores are based on a clinical population, the test was designed to only be utilized with individuals undergoing psychotherapy or psychological evaluation, it is not to be used for neurology purposes, in business, or to asses personality traits amongst a nonclinic-based population.

The MCMI-III utilizes base rate data rather than standard score transformations, such as T-scores. The goal of the MCMI-III is to generate profile patterns representative of clinical prevalence rates, and is therefore based on patients found to be disordered in diagnostic settings. As such, Base rate scores between 75 and 84 are considered subclinical and base rate scores above 85 are considered clinical, and more indicative of pathology. The Clinical Personality Patterns measured by MCMI-III are Avoidant, Depressive, Dependent, Histrionic, Narcissistic, Antisocial, Sadistic (Aggressive), Compulsive, Negativistic (Passive-Aggressive), and Masochistic (Self-Defeating). Schizotypal, Borderline, and Paranoid make up the Severe

Personality Pathology Scales. The Clinical Syndrome Scales encompass Anxiety, Somatoform, and Bipolar-Manic, Dysthymia, Alcohol Dependence, Drug Dependence, and Posttraumatic Stress Disorder. Thought Disorder, Major Depression, and Delusional Disorder and measured under the Severe Clinical Syndrome Scales.

The MCMI-III also utilizes four scales for evaluation of validity. The Validity Index (Scale V) consists of three highly improbable items. If two or more of these items are marked True, the protocol is invalid and a score of 1 indicates questionable validity. It is imperative that the clinician actually look at which items were marked true before determining invalidity as two of the questions could actually be marked True and reflect reality The Disclosure Index (Scale X) attempts to assess whether the individual was portraying open and honest answers or defensive and secretive answers. A raw score below 34 or above 178 indicates an invalid profile. The Debasement Index (Scale Y) measures whether the respondent was attempting to portray themselves in an overly favorable light, as not having any psychological difficulties. A Base Rate score over 75 on this measure shows a tendency to appear virtuous and the higher the score, the more they were not genuine. The Debasement Index (Scale Z) measures the respondent's attempt to portray themselves in a negative light, depreciating or devaluing themselves and endorsing more emotional difficulties. It is important to look at this score as it may indicate a cry for help when the respondent is severely emotionally distressed. When both the Desirability and Debasement scores are elevated, it indicates a patient who is self-disclosing in an unusual manner.

As far as PTSD, the MCMI-III introduced a specific scale to identify clinical characteristics. The overall profile pattern of elevated Avoidant and Passive-Aggressive scales were seen in male war veterans and female adult survivors of sexual and/or physical abuse.

Wisconsin Card Sorting Test (WCST)

The Wisconsin Card Sorting Test is used to assess executive functioning, namely the ability to shift and maintain problem-solving strategies for abstract problems when given feedback. The measure has been standardized for clients ages 6 ½ through 89 years of age. The test can be given by hand or with a computerized 128-card version. The client needs to match cards from a deck to one of four key cards based on an unknown sorting principle based upon feedback or "correct" or "incorrect." They are not told the strategy for sorting and must utilize the feedback to determine a response pattern. After a set number of correct responses, the sorting principal is changed, without the client being informed and they must generate a new hypothesis for their response pattern. Various scores are reported for the WCST including perseverative responses, number of trials to complete category 1, total number of trials, failure to maintain set, Percent Conceptual Level Responses. Perseverative errors occur when the examinee continues to respond to an incorrect characteristic. A failure to maintain set occurs when the examinee makes five or more correct consecutive matches but makes an error before completion of the category. Percent Conceptual Responses is utilized to measure insight into the correct sorting principle and shows consecutive correct responses, in a run of three or more.

Trail Making Test A and B

The Trail Making tests measure cognitive flexibility, set shifting, sequencing ability, visual-motor tracking, sequencing ability, and visual-motor speed. Trail A is a measure of visual scanning and motor speed. The examinee is asked to draw connecting lines between numbered circles in sequential order (1–2, 2–3, etc.). Trail B is similar to Trail A but also measures the ability to shift between different kinds of sequencing tasks. The examinee is asked to alternate between numbers and letters, in order, while connecting the circles (1 to A, 2 to B, 3 to C, etc.). Trails have an attentional component and are highly sensitive to the effects of brain injury.

Conners Continuous Performance Test III (CPT-III) and Conners Continuous Auditory Test of Attention (CATA)

The Conners Continuous Performance Test—III and Conners Continuous Auditory Test of Attention are computerized tests designed to assess symptoms of attention difficulties. The CPT-III is a visual measure to assess deficits in inattentiveness, impulsivity, sustained attention, and vigilance. The individual is instructed to response anytime a letter flashes on the screen, with the exception of the letter X. The test consists of 6 blocks, with 3 sub-blocks of 20 trials. Within each block, the stimulus is presented at different intervals (amount of time between presentations of each letter) over a 14 min time period. The CATA is an auditory measure utilized to assess deficits in inattentiveness, impulsivity, and sustained attention. The individual is instructed to respond when they hear a low tone, followed by a high tone and to not respond when they hear a high tone by itself.

A report is generated with a variety of scores to aid the clinician in determining the respondent's attentiveness. C measures the response style, conservative (accuracy over speed), liberal (speed over accuracy), or balanced (no bias to speed or accuracy). Response style should be taken into account during interpretation. D-prime measures the ability to detect between targets and non-targets. Omissions measures missed targets, not responding to stimuli and signals inattentiveness. Commissions occur when the respondent responds to non-targets and the reason for that response is indicated by the HRT (Hit Reaction Time) score. Therefore, elevated commission and slow reaction times lends itself to inattentiveness while elevated commission and fast reaction time indicates impulsivity. Perseverations occur when a response is made within 100 ms following a stimulus presentation, either the respondent reacted slowly to a previous stimulus, randomly responded, or attempted to anticipate the upcoming stimulus. Hit Reaction Time Standard Deviation assesses the consistency of response speed throughout the test. The higher the HRT SD< the more inconsistency which may indicate inattentiveness. Along those lines, HRT Block Change identifies the change in response time across the blocks of the test. A positive HRT signifies a slower response speed as the test progressed while a negative slope indicates faster response speed and a flat slope does not show any change. The report also provides an overall summary and clinical likelihood statement to aid in diagnosis. It is important that the examiner understand that a statement of very high, high, moderate, or minimal is only stating that the respondent has at least 1 symptom characterized by ADHD and must go on to interpret the individual dimensions of attention, inattentiveness, impulsivity, sustained attention, and vigilance.

Both the CPT-III and CATA are new versions of the CPT-II which have not been highly researched. Many in the field suggest that the CPT-II is still the better choice, and may be substituted instead of these newer versions until the value of the tests and their interpretive strategies have been clearly established.

Stroop Color-Word Test

The Stroop Color-Word Test is used to measure an individual's concentration and ability to switch between different kinds of cognitive tasks. The Stroop Test has three subtests, Word, Color, and Color-Word and each section is timed for 45 s. For the Word portion consists of the words Red, Green, and Blue arranged randomly and printed in black ink. The examinee is asked to read aloud, as quickly as possible, the words on the page, completing each column. The Color portion consists of 100 items, written as XXXX, printed in Green, Blue, or Red ink. The examinee is required to read the color of ink the XXXX is printed in, as quickly as possible. The Color-Word portion consists of the words from the Word page printed in the colors from the Color page and the examinee is asked to quickly read aloud the color of ink the word is printed in, not the word itself. The Stroop generates a wide array of clinical data, with higher scores generally reflecting better performance. On the Interference score, low scores, below 40 indicate difficulties, but high scores, like those acquired by someone with dyslexia because they have low reading scores, are indicative of a lack of interference. The Stroop can help identify reading disabilities, brain injuries to left parietal-temporal areas, lack of motivation, and prefrontal disorders.

Minnesota Multiphasic Personality Inventory 2 (MMPI-2)

The Minnesota Multiphasic Personality Inventory 2 is an assessment that elicits a wide range of self-descriptions scored to give a quantitative measurement of an individual's level of emotional adjustment and attitude toward test taking. The norms are based on data from adult men and women from various ethnic groups and racial minority groups representing several geographic regions of the United States. The MMPI-2 requires a sixth-grade level of reading comprehension. The most commonly used scores from the measure consist of validity scales and the 10 clinical scales. A multitude of additional scales and interpretations are available, but for brevity are unable to be discussed here.

The Validity scales consist of measures of inconsistent responding, infrequent responding, and measures of defensiveness. The VRIN (Variable Response Inconsistency) scale is used to determine if the respondent answered in a consistent fashion to items with similar content. TRIN (True Response Inconsistency) scale is used to determine how a respondent answers to items consisting of opposite content. The F (Infrequency) Scale measures the amount of responses to infrequent items that were endorsed. The Fb (Back F) Scale attempts to measure infrequent responding to the back half of the test to determine if the respondent's attitude or test taking approach changed over the course of the test. The L (Lie) Scale and K (Correction) scales are utilized to measure defensiveness. The L scale considers if the test taker approaches the measure in a defensive manner, denying minor faults and character flaws that many persons are willing to admit about themselves. The K scale measures defensiveness in responding and attempts to correct for this response style on clinical scales (Butcher et al. 2001).

The 10 clinical scales consist of Hypochondriasis (Hs), Depression (D), Hysteria (HY), Psychopathic Deviate (Pd), Masculinity-Femininity (Mf), Paranoia (Pa), Psychasthenia (Pt), Schizophrenia (Sc), Hypomania (Ma), and Social Introversion (Si). The Hypochondriasis scale attempts to measure respondents who express an excessive concern regarding health and present with somatic complaints that do not have a basis for physical diagnosis. They tend to have bodily preoccupation and self-centered focus. Elevations on the Depression scale indicate feelings of dysphoria, hopelessness, and pessimism. Item content also encapsulates somatic complaints, difficulties controlling ones' thoughts, and worry. The 60 items of the Hysteria scale encompass physical complaints, and denial of life problems and social anxiety. The Psychopathic Deviate scale is meant to measure difficulties with authority, lack of concern for others, lowered moral standards, and familial problems. The Masculinity–Femininity scale covers a wide array of items including work, worries, fears, sensitivity, family relationships, and work. The scale tends to identify males or females tendency to conform to or reject traditional stereotypical gender roles. The Paranoia scale consists of items focused on psychotic behaviors and symptoms moral concerns, sensitivity, and how they deal with other people. The Psychasthenia scale looks to focus on worries, anxiety, compulsions, and fears, with the modern label leaning toward obsessive compulsive disorder. The Schizophrenia scale originally attempted to tease out symptoms of different types of schizophrenia, however was unsuccessful and the current scale focuses on psychotic symptoms, bizarre mentation, hallucinations, peculiarities, family relationships, and social concerns. The Hypomania scale was designed to capture symptoms of hypomania including grandiosity, activity level, and excitability. Family concerns, morals, and bodily concerns are also covered within this scale. Finally, The Social Introversion scale attempts to

measure social introversion and extroversion. The questions focus on social participation and neurotic maladjustment (Butcher et al. 2001).

With regards to PTSD, the PK (Posttraumatic Stress Disorder-Keane) Scale
(found in Content Scales) attempts to identify the disorder in war veterans and was
normed with scores from Vietnam combat veterans. High scores on this scale endorse
anxiety, sleep disturbance, fear of losing emotional and/or cognitive control,
disturbing thoughts, and intense emotional distress. Prior studies, based on the
MMPI, had identified 2-8/8-2 as a PTSD profile, but this has not been as widely
replicated on the MMPI-2, and it is thought to believe that high elevations on Scale
7 have caused this change (Lyons and Wheeler-Cox 1999). Unfortunately, the available literature does not lend itself to discussion of TBI profiles in the MMPI-2, rather
it focuses on validity, malingering, and civil litigation. This is a hole in the literature
and interesting topic for research.

Chapter 4
Interpretation

As can be seen from the previous material, there is no simple formula for separating TBI and PTSD in many cases. Interpretation requires a rigorous integration of information from history, neuropsychological testing, psychological testing, neurological results, neuroradiological results, and generally medical information which can reasonably impact any of the above factors. The accuracy of the information obtained is essential to the accuracy of the diagnosis and the diagnostic formulation. This applies not only to the psychological and neuropsychological testing as previously described but also to the history and medical information.

In many cases seen by the authors, diagnostic errors have arisen because much of the history has been distorted because evaluator chose to rely on a client's own recall as to the sequence of events and the events themselves or relied on secondary sources that wrote down what the patient told them (which does not give the statement more factual accuracy). When primary sources are retrieved, the actual information is very different from that told by the client. This may not be malingering: the client may very well believe what he or she says is true, but they be wrong because they misunderstood, because they are repeating what someone else surmised, or they have distorted their own memories to fit in with a storyline which gives them comfort or which absolves them of blame or guilt. However, if we rely on this information, we fall into a trap of diagnosing what they want us to diagnose rather than what we should be looking for.

For example, the senior author had one case in which a young girl was hit by a car as a pedestrian. She was apparently hit while walking along the side of the road by an object that was of the shape of a truck side view mirror, and sent flying through the air, severely injuring her head with extensive intra-cranial bleeding. The truck did not stop and perhaps may not even have known they hit her. Her body was found by a jogger who called 911 and she was rushed into neurosurgery. She had extensive

© The Author(s) 2016

C.J. Golden et al., *The Intercorrelation of Traumatic Brain Injury and PTSD in Neuropsychological Evaluations*, SpringerBriefs in Behavioral Criminology, DOI 10.1007/978-3-319-47033-7_4

blood loss along with the severe brain injury but survived. She was in a coma for several weeks and when she became aware she had no memory for what had happened and for several weeks prior. She improved in terms of speech and IQ but her memory for the events prior to the injury for several weeks and after the injury for several weeks showed no improvement.

A friend expressed to her the belief that she did not believe that she was randomly injured by a passing vehicle and that something more serious had occurred. In talking, they began to speculate she had been attacked and raped. Over time, the girl started to dream that she had been raped. This dream became more vivid over time and the client started to have PTSD like symptoms including fear of men who approached her. Within a year she was diagnosed with PTSD due to a rape.

The problem with this was that her story—which eventually came out in vivid detail—was totally inconsistent with the known facts of the case. She remembered she had been grabbed, her blouse ripped off, and then she was thrown to the ground and her bra ripped off and her breasts fondled. Then her pants had been removed and her underpants ripped, followed by penetration and then she was hit on the head. The difficulty with the story is that when she was found she was fully clothed. There were some tears in her outer clothing consistent with being hit by the truck and thrown to the ground, but her bra and underpants were completely intact and there was no evidence of penetration or rape. Despite the evidence against her story, she became more firmly convinced of the truth of her story and it became more embellished over time and more serious. She started in therapy with a therapist who believed her whole story, seeing this purely as PTSD. The therapy resulted in further reinforcing her belief that she had been raped and "someone important" was covering it up to protect someone else. It should be noted that she never recovered any accurate or verifiable memories of what had occurred for several weeks before the accident. In addition to the obvious problem of believing a story which could not be true, this case also illustrates the role of TBI, through a frontal injury, in predisposing someone towards the developing PTSD despite no real memory of an event, through the disruption of the ability to perceive reality and control emotional lability.

Other common errors in history are exaggerations of the severity of the head injury one has suffered. Early information is important because the symptoms of TBI generally improve over time and are at the worst in the immediate period after the injury, with severable notable exceptions: (1) when edema builds up in the brain (like an ankle swelling) causing high pressure which if not treated can lead to an increase of symptoms over a period of up to several weeks. This may also occur when hematomas develop; (2) The brain is not injured by the accident but by injuries to the cardiac, respiratory, or other bodily systems which over time impact the brain as well; (3) Seizures develop which are of sufficient magnitude to further injure the brain or interfere with its operations; and (4) there are subsequent neurological or medical events following the first event but which are unrelated. However, when more serious cognitive symptoms develop over time these are more likely be due to emotional and environmental factors. These factors can include delayed PTSD symptoms where the event memories come back more clearly over time and then in turn display an impact on the reported cognitive symptoms. They can also include other environmental factors such as anger on the person seen as the cause of the injury, anger on the insurance company or hospital involved, anger on the family for not supporting them as they see appropriate, or frustration from failure due to returning to work or school too early before complete resolution of any acute symptoms. Another related and more insidious factor arises when a psychologist or other professional gives early tests or just opinions and overinterprets the results as permanent brain damage, setting up expectations for failure and decline. This is not uncommon in our litigious society when an individual with a minor head trauma seen primarily for an orthopedic or pain injury goes to a lawyer and is sent to the lawyer's psychologist who adds brain damage as a diagnosis even though there was no previous evidence for such a diagnosis. Sometime this is an insightful discovery but it is often the result of poorly interpreted (and administered) data.

This leads us to the last area in which history plays an important role: the relationship between TBI severity and TBI symptoms. Since in most states, psychologists are allowed to give neuropsychological tests with little or no training (as do some neurologists and psychiatrists as well), there has developed a subset of neuropsychological interpretation that recognizes any deficit in any test as brain damage. Since we all have weaknesses and strengths—as previously discussed—almost everyone has some relative deficit, give enough tests of sufficient breadth and complexity. Other deficits will arise because of motivational levels, effort, how seriously the tests are taken, and the presence of other non-neuropsychological disorders. Thus, interpretation must be more sophisticated and focus on how consistent the testing is with, what is reasonably expected for a given disorder, and the individuals' premorbid level of functioning.

This requires a neuropsychological interpretation which allows for the integration of the known effects of a given disorder and the medical history of the individual combined with an understanding of how the complex brain works. Some of these cases are simple: An individual with a mild head injury with only brief loss of consciousness and no complications tested as having a fifty point drop in IQ, an impossible result from that disorder, suggesting either malingering or that the observed drop was due to other factors such as PTSD or Major Depression. In another case, a bus driver was sent back to work after testing, after a very minor head injury with no known complications. Testing revealed a highly focal right parietal lesion—an MRI identified a tumor that of course was not caused by the accident, but which likely caused it.

There is a wealth of the literature on the effects of different disorders, the impact on different locations in the brain, and the impact across age groups and across levels of premorbid achievement. For the purpose of this volume, however, the major interests are those factors which impact the cognitive expression of TBI. When trying to understand a differentiation between PTSD and TBI, an understanding of these factors is essential in judging which disorder one is looking at.

TBIs can be subclassified on many dimensions. One of the most basic is whether a disorder is a penetrating (open) head injury or simply a closed (non-penetrating injury). A penetrating injury is indicated when the skull is broken through such that the brain itself is directly damaged by the penetrating object such as a bullet, shrapnel, iron bar, wooden stake, or any other object capable of penetrating through the skull and into the brain. In general, people call any injury which fractures the skull, a penetrating injury although neuropsychologically the issue is not whether the skull is penetrated but whether the penetration reaches the brain itself. In cases where only the skull is fractured but the brain is not, these can act more like a closed head injury with the force communicated to the brain actually reduced by the fracturing of the skull.

In penetrating injuries, the effects of the head injury are generally more focal, corresponding to those areas of the brain which are destroyed by the penetrating object or by the fragments of the skull being pushed into the brain tissue. Localized damage is also caused by rupturing of the vascular or cerebral spinal fluid systems, whose fluids cause further localized damage. Damage to the vascular system can also disrupt blood flow to areas of the brain when the vascular system is interrupted. These latter areas may be significantly removed from the areas of the original injury. In more severe cases such injuries will often result in death.

Penetrating injuries will also traumatize the brain causing edema resulting in a swelling of the brain. Such swelling causes increases in the pressure within the brain which can compress and damage brain tissue as well as make it harder—if not impossible—for the heart to maintain blood flow to the brain, resulting in hypoxia, anoxia, and even death. Depending on the degree of loss of the skull (which contains the swelling and causes the pressure) the pressure may not increase as much as in a closed head injury although the degree to which there is any significant opening in the skull is generally limited in those cases which survive, as any injury resulting in a large fragmentation of the skull is also more likely to result in death or extreme injuries such as vegetative states.

Closed head injuries are most often the result of the force of an object or explosion being transmitted through the skull to the brain, with the degree of transmission depending on several factors. These include the ability of the skull to absorb part of the force, as well as the relevant movement of the head to the object impacting the skull. For example, if we can drop bowling ball directly down on a head such that the head cannot move, the impact is greater than if the same force moves laterally and the head moves away from the direction of the force. In some of the injuries, while the initial force may look impressive, the ability of the head to move quickly enough (depending on the speed of the force) may make hitting the ground a more significant factor than the original force. This applies not only to forces caused by actual objects but also blast forces which can be just as deadly as a car accident or being hit with a baseball bat.

A subtype of closed head injury is acceleration–deceleration injuries. These injuries are most often caused not by a force directly applied to the brain, but by sudden stops in the speed of the head caused in car accidents or other transportation or objects that move, and may, in theory, also be caused by sudden deceleration. This type of injury may occur in concert with impacting another object or simply as a restrained sudden stop.

These injuries can create focal effects at the point of contact by an object (where the force is transmitted directly to the brain tissue below the contact point) or to the opposite point in the brain where the force causes the brain to shift away from the force impacting the skull on the opposite side (called coup-counter-coup) or causes the skull to move away from the force at a different speed than the brain causing injury when there is a subsequent impact between the brain and the skull causing a focal injury. The speed at which these collisions occur determines the possible focal impacts.

Most often closed head injuries have more diffuse effects than focal effects. These can arise through axonal shearing where the longer axons within the brain are stretched out through the movement of the head, impacting those skills which are dependent on complex interactions across the brain (for example, memory, concentration, higher level assessment of novel situations), but much less so on those which depend on shorter axonal connections (such as speech or reading or other well practiced skills).

However, not all closed head injuries are this simple. These injuries may be accompanied by complications, most often edema and bleeding. As noted above, edema causes the brain to swell. Since the brain is constrained by the skull, this causes an increase in pressure within the brain. If severe enough, such pressure increases can impair blood flow to the brain, resulting in hypoxia or anoxia until the pressure is relieved either on its own (such as the improvement of selling in any other part of the body), by medication, or, in some cases, by removing part of the skull so that the brain may expand without the normal constrictions of the skull. All edema does not cause long-term effects, even when short-term effects such as changes in consciousness, memory problems, incontinence, concentration problems, balance problems, and papilledema.

Bleeding occurs most often as hematomas, often in the subdural area of the brain, as well as bleeding in the brain itself or occasional rupturing of the cerebral spinal system. Subdural hematomas (and similar conditions) are space occupying lesions which arise from bleeding into the subdural space of the meninges due to ruptures of the vessels which attach the brain to the meninges. While these vessels can rupture in anyone at any age, such ruptures can occur more easily in older individuals where the shrinking normal brain actually hangs from the meninges by these blood vessels as opposed to younger individuals where the brain normally fits snugly within the skull and the meninges.

While hematomas sound serious, they create problems only when they increase pressure within the brain to a point where these are actual damage to the brain from compression or, as with edema, blood flow is restricted. Many hematomas remain small and reabsorb or become static on their own and have no effects on cognitive or emotional functions. More dangerous hematomas which continue to grow can be drained by surgical intervention if the individual receives prompt and appropriate medical care. Only when the hematoma continues to grow without intervention to a dangerous size do they become an issue. For example, the senior author saw an elderly Professor at a major University who was injured in what appeared to be a minor bicycle accident with just some scrapes and bruises and no loss of consciousness. He went home and went to sleep. Twelve hours later he was found unconscious as a result of an unchecked hematoma which caused severe hypoxia. While he did

not die, he lost over fifty IQ points from his premorbid levels and never again func-
tioned independently. Had he stayed awake and went to a hospital with a headache
which would have accompanied the increasing pressure, he could have been treated
surgically and had no ill effects.

Other bleeding occurs within the brain itself as a result of the rupture of brain
vessels secondary to the force of the blow. This bleeding can arise from any size
vessels from small capillaries whose bleeding may not be serious to major arteries
where the symptoms will look more like a major or minor stroke than a head injury.
In other cases, these major ruptures occur in a pre-existing weak spot (aneurysm/
malformation) in a vessel, or occur in a vessel which has been weakened by arte-
riosclerosis or other disease process. The impact of this bleeding is determined by
the degree and scope of the bleeding as it would in any stroke process. These disorders can create anywhere from very mild and unimportant lasting deficits to severe
losses. One young woman seen for evaluation had a mild head injury and developed
headaches, quickly followed by hemiparesis. It was discovered at the hospital that
she had a massive malformation of the vascular system which encompassed nearly
half of the right cerebral hemisphere and which started bleeding an increasing rate
after the trauma. Her symptoms, as in the case of all of these bleeding disorders, are
based on the location and size and appear as localized lesions.

One last comment on the medical evidence used to diagnose all of these disorders,
which heavily rely on results from CT scans and MRIs, as well as other neuroradiological devices. While many of these conditions are obvious on CTs and MRIs down
contemporaneously with an accident, others ranging from hematomas which may
grow in periods of hours to weeks to the long term impact of axonal shearing and
edema which may not be seen for months or years as unusual brain atrophy after the
death of neurons. There are cases where medical evidence is initially missing, but
historical and neuropsychological details suggest that something is there which was
missed. In such cases, later evaluations can be very useful in determining whether
such symptoms have a true medical cause or are the result of lack of effort or
emotional issues.

Injuries get Better. Emotional Conditions may get worse. A basic tenet of
assessment for these disorders is that over time TBI the symptoms of TBI get better
(barring medical complications or another injury) or stay the same, while the symptoms of PTSD may get worse over time. This does not mean that people who get
worse do not have a TBI, but it usually indicates that additional symptoms such as
increased memory loss, concentration problems, and the like are more likely the
result of the emotional issues involved rather than the original TBI. The assessor
must keep in mind however that some symptoms of TBI may not show up if not
measured or observed: Concentration may be okay in a structured (and boring)
hospital setting, but not adequate when returning to work or school. The evaluators'
job is made much easier when neuropsychological testing precedes sending the client
back into the community.

It is recognized that, in many settings, a full testing battery as described here is
not possible. In such cases a screening battery can be employed, ideally one that
focuses on more complex functions rather than tests like the Mini Mental Status

Exam or computerized tests aimed at looking at the immediate, acute effects of TBI. A possible abbreviated battery from the tests suggested here can consist of Matrices, Visual Puzzles and Symbol Search from the WAIS-IV, Visual Reproduction from the WMS-IV, the Stroop Color and Word Test, WRAT Reading, and the Trail Making Test. These require minimal equipment and can be given in under an hour in a hospital or outpatient setting. The screening battery offers good estimates of premorbid IQ (Matrices, Reading) as well as measured which are sensitive to complex and basic impairment arising from TBI. If scores are abnormal, this indicates the need for more comprehensive assessment.

The longer one waits to get an initial baseline, the more one is unable to make a reasonable assessment of the etiology of specific symptoms, which may occur as a result of emotional, medical, or personal stressors unrelated to brain injury. One must be suspect of symptoms of TBI which are significantly delayed from the onset of the disorder and those which deteriorate over time.

On the other hand, emotional symptom may get worse over time as the person better recalls the event from their own memory or from the second-hand accounts of others. PTSD is also clearly known to have a delayed component in some clients as their attempts to suppress or deny the symptoms may fail over time. Other factors, such as survivor guilt, the delayed death of others involved in the event, poor support or interactions with support systems and loss of job or school failure may also enhance these symptoms.

As noted earlier, a good and detailed history as to when symptoms started is essential. This often needs to include interviews with significant others as early as possible in the course of the disorder as clients may be inaccurate, in denial, or lack insight. (giving standardized tests, such as the MMPI-2, does not make up for inaccurate results arising from a lack of insight of one's own symptoms). Interviews must insist on specifics of what behaviors are impaired rather than accepting generalities and conclusions that someone is depressed or anxious or any other similar symptoms.

Litigation. Not surprisingly, the introduction of litigation into the process can have a negative impact on the assessment, as the litigation itself represents a new stressor and introduces secondary gain as a possible motivator. Litigation here is broadly defined not only as criminal or civil suits arising from an incident but also applications for such things as disability or accommodations at work or school. This can lead to individuals being less than truthful about preexisting deficits as well as exaggeration of symptoms. Psychologists themselves may fall into a role of advocate rather than evaluator which colors one's entire evaluation, sometimes conscious but also unconsciously in a desire to help a client in distress or in the real word to get more referrals from a given source. It is incumbent on the evaluator to try and stay neutral with a focus on accuracy rather than what a client or attorney wants you to find.

In doing an assessment in these conditions, it is important not only to look at data supportive of your conclusions but also to focus on all the data which contradicts your conclusions and to address both sides in your evaluation. (In civil or criminal litigation the assessor should also clearly let the attorney and/or client know both sides of the issue so they may proceed in the most effective manner). Reports for disability or accommodations should clearly outline the pros and cons of a specific accommodation or the impact of deficits on disability considerations.

Effort. Clearly related to litigation issues and concerns over test validity and the accuracy of the history are the questions related to motivation and effort. Psychologists tend to assume that everyone they see is putting in maximum effort and wish to do their very best on testing. This is frequently not the case. The lack of motivation and effort may range from those who consciously wish to deceive (malingering) to those who simply are uninterested in cooperating. In other cases, they may begin a test with effort but quickly become frustrated and uncooperative. While malingering tests may pick out the former, individuals who become easily frustrated may do well on malingering tests which are relatively easy.

Those with high levels of frustration either because of a TBI or PTSD usually can be identified only by close observation. Their behavior during testing is mercurial and they overreact to signs they have failed which are embedded in the test (e.g., Category Test or Block Design) or from their own perception (accurate or not) that they are doing poorly. Some clients faced with evidence of failure redouble their efforts to succeed; others complain and give up. In the latter case, their scores are unlikely to reflect their real abilities. Such individuals need frequent praise and support as well as encouragement to go beyond the imaginary limits they have set for themselves.

Individuals with effort problems will often show scores inconsistent with their day-to-day functioning, an important observation they may indicate the need to readminister a test or to use an alternate test of the same function. In other cases, some tests may show unusual scores more than 1.5 standard deviations from their average score which may require reconsideration of the validity of that score. In making comparisons of scores, it is important to measure scores only against similar scores—for example, look at the deviation of a verbal score from other verbal scores. Not all deviant scores are inaccurate, but clear consideration needs to be given to such scores in this population.

Individuals who are deliberately or unconsciously putting in maximum effort may be more likely seen using traditional tests of malingering. Generally, these tests can be seen as either tests of behavioral and personality malingering, and tests of cognitive malingering. The most common personality malingering tests are often embedded with such tests as the MMPI-2 or MCMI-III. Currently, the most respected stand-alone tests are the SIRS, which was discussed in the previous chapter.

There are a large number of cognitive effort tests like the TOMM which was discussed previously. One should keep in mind however that a test of memory malingering, like the TOMM, may not reflect lowered effort in individuals whose malingering is in executive tests. There must be care taken to avoid overgeneralization of the meaning of these scores.

In individuals who have had multiple tests, unexplained inconsistencies may be indications of inadequate effort especially when scores drop over time without a reasonable neuropsychological explanation. In such cases, using their highest score is most often the best estimate of their ability, although even that score may be an underestimate. In cases where scores increase over time, test–retest effects must be considered. However, such an effect is unlikely if the original performance was very poor. For example, if someone fails to complete any categories on the Wisconsin Card Sort Test, it is unlikely they learned anything from the test; therefore, a later change cannot be attributed to test–retest effects. However, if they completed three or fours categories, a jump to six later may not be surprising. Similarly, on Memory tests, a jump from poor performance two standard deviations below the mean to an average score cannot be attributed to prior learning or a test–retest effect.

Diagnostic Choices Between PTSD and TBI

As PTSD and TBI are not mutually exclusive, we have basically four diagnostic choices: (1) Neither is present; (2) Only TBI is present; (3) Only PTSD is present; and (4) Both are present.

Neither are Present. This is the easiest of the diagnostic choices: the individual fails to meet the criteria for either disorder as discussed here. Any trauma present was mild and recovered within two to three months. Any initial anxiety symptoms have decreased and do not interfere with day-to-day activities. Oddly, this diagnostic combination is seen frequently in litigation cases before litigation has begun—after the beginning of litigation, reported symptoms increase. While this is possible with PTSD symptoms, TBI symptoms (as previously noted) will improve unless there has been a medical complication of some kind. It is always important to note that some TBI symptoms may be masked initially by keeping the individual out of school or work in cases where there is a new onset of symptoms which are delayed, immediate testing is necessary to establish a baseline and to be balanced against expectations from the injury via the history.

TBI only. *Most* TBI clients do not initially report symptoms of PTSD as their primary symptoms, so diagnosis is rather clear cut initially. Individuals clearly must meet the criteria for a TBI as previously discussed, and symptoms may range from mild to severe. Moderate and severe cases of TBI are usually easily observed and confirmed by neurological or neuropsychological testing. Milder cases can be missed initially, but most will recover within 3–6 months with or without identification. Few of these cases will develop PTSD as described earlier because the event themselves are generally not remembered and do not have the impact on psychological functioning (described below) that is seen in real PTSD.

TBI clients are more likely to develop depression, anger, and frustration as result of an inability to deal with their losses arising from cognitive impairment or physical losses. While they will often blame this on the accident involved (or on the legal process if they are involved), they will not show typical symptoms which would indicate PTSD, although their focus on the accident may result in an inappropriate diagnosis of PTSD.

PTSD only. In the absence of TBI, PTSD is seen primarily as an emotional disorder. However, it is well known that clients with PTSD with no history of a possible TBI or neurological injury often show cognitive symptoms which are indicative of a brain disorder (as may be seen in other major pathologies as well). To understand the neuropsychological connection here, one must examine the cognitive structure of the brain.

The brain can be divided into three major units, which can be further subdivided but that is unnecessary for this discussion. The three units consist of: (1) the subcortical areas of the brain, which play a major role in emotion, memory, attention, and sensorimotor functions; (2) the posterior of the brain, including most of the temporal, parietal and occipital lobes, which processes sensory information and is responsible for understanding speech, visual-spatial functions, academic functions, and intellectual functions as measured by traditional psychometric tests; and (3) the anterior of the brain (frontal lobes and parts of the temporal lobe) which coordinate motor functions and output, but, more importantly, are responsible for higher level executive functions, which include such processes as emotional regulation, planning, organization, evaluation, flexibility, insight, emotional maturity, restraint, and all those functions which separate a bright 12 year old from a mature adult.

From a neuropsychological perspective, the traditional view of PTSD (begun by a serious trauma), indicates the initial impact is on the first unit of the brain. This area is responsible for our most basic biological emotional reactions. The degree of reaction is not the same in everyone: emotional reactivity is influences by one's genetics which determine a person's basic temperament, modified by a lifetime of learning. This area of the brain is relative primitive, focused on survival (fight or flight), identifying those stimuli which are a threat to the organism and subject to one-trial Pavlovian learning in intense situations. In extreme situations, this area will overreact, but usually over time calm down when the threat is removed (or the organism is exhausted).

When the organism is threatened, the subcortical area send impulses to the third unit of the brain in order to commence more complex responses to the situation than the reflexive and automatic responses which can arise from the first unit of the brain. In ideal circumstances, these impulses initiate appropriate motor and cognitive responses to handle the emergency situation. In some cases, these impulses become overwhelming, disrupting the functions of the frontal lobe, and leading to cognitive paralysis or inappropriate reactions.

PTSD occurs in situations when these impulses from the subcortical areas do not cease after the completion of the event as would normally be expected. This can occur for several reasons. The most obvious is that the trauma is so severe that the normal "calming" process fails to take place. It is clear however that this is an individualized process: when faced with the same event, some people will develop PTSD and others will not. This can be due to a lower physiological threshold for some people due simply to their genetic inheritance or due to past experience.

However, PTSD from a neuropsychological prospective may occur not as a result of the function of the subcortical areas, but as a result of the function of the third unit of the brain. In all situations, including trauma, the third unit of the brain may act to exacerbate or lessen an emotional reaction. Exacerbation may occur because of a pessimistic attitude or hopelessness or a catastrophic reaction that is cognitive rather than emotional in nature. Exacerbation may occur because the third unit is overwhelmed by the incoming stimuli and be unable to deal with them. Just as there are ascending tracks communicating from the first unit of the brain to the third unit, there are descending neural tracks which allow the third unit to dampen or exacerbate the emotional reactions within the first unit. These downward connections can act to maintain an emotional reaction or even exacerbate the emotional reaction. In such cases, the maintenance or exacerbation causes additional stimuli to rise up from the first unit to the third unit, causing in turn more impulses to be sent back, creating a "vicious circle" which feeds upon itself. External pressures (such as a lawsuit or a reluctance or inability to return to work or school), feelings of guilt for survival, financial issues, and other related factors may also influence how the third unit affects the functions of the first unit.

On the positive side, the third unit ideally acts not to exacerbate but reduce the emotional stimuli. Higher cognitive processes may be used to reduce the functioning in the first unit, avoiding the "vicious circle" described above. One of the major functions of the third unit is to inhibit impulses arising from the first unit ("maturity") so we gain more emotional control as the third unit fully develops from ages 12–15. Just as we can talk ourselves into overreaction, we can talk ourselves into underreaction. By minimizing the cognitive reactions to events or to strong emotional stimuli, the development of PTSD can be avoided in cases where the frontal areas remain in control and not overwhelmed. This ability of the higher cognitive areas to control the emotional areas of the brain is responsible for the success of some cognitive/verbal interventions to lessen the symptoms of PTSD, although some experiential/visualization may be necessary to fully reduce some of the conditioned emotional responses to specific stimuli involved in the development of the PTSD.

Visualization also plays a role in the development of PTSD. Exacerbation of the underlying emotional stimuli can be caused by reliving the events involved in the trauma, which requires not only the subcortical memory areas, but also the participation of the second and third units of the brain. These memories may arise through direct stimulation by the emotional areas and/or by triggering stimuli, but also through the cognitive areas of the brain which can also focus on reliving the event and further exacerbating the emotional response. It should be noted that the memories themselves may be misinterpreted and modified by these higher brain areas, both in ways that make the event worse and in ways that lessen the impact of these areas.

The cognitive symptoms seen in PTSD arise from the strong stimuli from the first unit of the brain which interferes with cognitive processes in both the second and third units of the brain. In addition, the third unit itself can disrupt even basic cognitive processes in the second unit of the brain. This can arise to the level where it appears that a head injury has occurred, with testing showing extensive impairment. Such testing however is inconsistent of the absence of a known brain injury or greatly exaggerated from what would be expected in a mild, unseen injury. This is complicated, however, by the fact that this can occur in cases with real brain injuries as well, with the presentation being greatly exaggerated by these processes despite the presence of a real injury. As noted previously, however, the real head injury symptoms will generally be evident early on rather than the more severe deficits which arise later. Clearly, early evaluation and attention to the balance of cognitive and emotional symptoms is important to diagnosis, and likely to treatment as well.

Both are present. The key issues here are cases where the brain injury occurs before or at the same time of the PTSD-related trauma, although acquisition of a brain injury at a later time can exacerbate the preexisting PTSD using the same mechanisms described here. In general, the presence of a brain injury influences the relationship between the first and third unit through injury to the ascending or descending connections or through injuries to the first or third brain units themselves.

In theory, injuries to just the ascending tracks—which send impulses from the first unit to the third unit—should actually lessen the chance of the development of PTSD. Such a hypothetical injury would prevent the emotional impulses from rising to the third unit and avoiding the disruption discussed previously on cognitive functions and avoiding the loop which results in PTSD. In fact, the theory behind frontal lobotomies which disconnected the first and third units of the brain lessen emotional reactivity and the interference of emotions on cognition and voluntary behavior. Such operations are not a good idea as they turn out to have many serious side effects while reportedly achieving the goal of disconnection.

Injuries to the descending tracks from the third unit to the first unit would also interrupt the "vicious circle" described above, but would not avoid the frontal lobes being overwhelmed by the impulses arising from the first unit of the brain. It would also not avoid the cognitive disruption of the second unit caused by the first unit, or possible indirect effects of the second unit on the third unit which are normally not important in adult disorders.

In most cases, the injuries which occur do not destroy these tracks but rather cause stretching of neurons and interfere with the interfaces between endings of axons and dendrites on the connecting neuron, with the effects being strongest with longer axonal connections and at the cortical–subcortical interfaces. This does not eliminate the connections, but slows down their transmission and makes the connections unreliable and inaccurate. This has a lesser effect on the ascending tracks which are generally sending messages of danger, anxiety, or depression with relatively little content, while the descending tracks attempt to control and modify these more primitive areas show more impact. Thus, the result is the continuation of the emotional symptoms upward without the ability to dampen these impulses, leading to a higher chance of the development of PTSD. Such a situation would also make the use of verbal-based therapies less effective as the frontal lobes would be reduced in their ability to mitigate the emotional reactions.

Injuries to the third unit of the brain have in general an amplifying effect on the course of PTSD. Third unit injuries may not show any obvious intellectual deficits and may not even show motor deficits, but will still interfere with higher level cognitive processes. Primary among these processes are the ability to inhibit the first unit of the brain and to deal effectively with the impulses arising from the first unit. When faced with impulses from the first unit, the injured frontal lobes may deal with them ineffectively, causing more cognitive disorganization. In turn, even if the impulses are processed effectively, the ability to inhibit and control the first unit is lessened. If either of these conditions or both are present, there is an increased likelihood that PTSD symptoms will be developed and maintained, as well as an increased inability to respond to therapy. In addition, the injured frontal lobe may misinterpret memories in such a way as to enhance the negative effects of the situation. (It can also misinterpret in a manner which decreases the negative effects or fails to acknowledge the situation at all, but this clearly does not result in PTSD symptomatology). The inability of the person to deal cognitively with the impulses from the first unit and to adapt can also lead to frustration and depression at the cognitive level, leading further to an exacerbation of the symptoms. Overall, injuries to the third unit clearly enhance the likelihood of PTSD while at the same time decreasing responses to therapy.

Injuries to the first unit of the brain may also enhance the likelihood of PTSD. These permanent injuries are more common from penetrating head wounds than from closed TBI or blast injuries. Injuries can cause an enhancement of negative emotions and flooding of the brain with these feelings, resulting in even smaller events taking on greater emotional stimuli. TBI can temporarily interfere with the formation of new memories, which should in theory interfere with the development of PTSD as the person is unaware of the events involved. This works in many TBI patients; however, in some cases, the patient forms false memories from the reports of doctors and people they know or written reports and "regain" memories which in turn lead to PTSD. Such a situation is made more likely when the frontal lobes are injured as well which leads to misperception of what is experientially real and what is learned from other sources. In rare cases, seizures in the emotional areas develop which lead to very strong or overwhelming feelings of depression, anxiety, or fear. When this occurs, the brain tries to explain the feelings and may focus on a specific event or trauma, resulting in PTSD, or may focus on individuals or organizations, resulting in paranoia. These seizures can often be treated effectively with medication.

Conclusions

Overall, there is a complex interplay between TBI and PTSD, sometimes to a point where they are difficult to distinguish from one another. TBI especially may enhance the likelihood and severity of PTSD, except in cases where the loss of memory results in an inability to relive the event, although false memories may be substituted in the normal or injured brain. Separation of the conditions is made easier by early comprehensive evaluations and thorough and accurate histories. Correlation with the known effects of brain injuries and the results of neuroradiological tests is important but not absolute as there are many exceptions which need to be considered. An understanding of these causes and their interaction is considered essential to good treatment planning and expectations.

References

Alexander, M. P. (1995). Mild traumatic brain injury: Pathophysiology, natural history, and clinical management. *Neurology, 45*(7), 1253–1260.

American Psychiatric Association. (1994). *Diagnostic and statistical manual of mental disorders: DSM- IV* (4th ed.). Washington, DC: American Psychiatric Association.

American Psychiatric Association. (2000). *Diagnostic and statistical manual of mental disorders: DSM-IV-TR*. Washington, DC: American Psychiatric Association.

American Psychiatric Association. (2013). *Diagnostic and statistical manual of mental disorders* (5th ed.). Arlington, VA: American Psychiatric Publishing.

Ashman, T. A., Spielman, L. A., Hibbard, M. R., Silver, J. M., Chandna, T., & Gordon, W. A. (2004). Psychiatric challenges in the first 6 years after traumatic brain injury: Cross-sequential analyses of Axis I disorders. *Archives of Physical Medicine and Rehabilitation, 85*, 36–42.

Barrow, I. M., Hough, M., Rastatter, M. P., Walker, M., Holbert, D., & Rotondo, M. F. (2006). The effects of mild traumatic brain injury on confrontation naming in adults. *Brain Injury, 20* (8), 845–855.

Belanger, H. G., Curtiss, G., Demery, J. A., Lebowitz, B. K., & Vanderploeg, R. D. (2005). Factors moderating neuropsychological outcomes following mild traumatic brain injury: A meta-analysis. *Journal of the International Neuropsychological Society, 11*(03), 215–227.

Belanger, H. G., Kretzmer, T., Vanderploeg, R. D., & French, L. M. (2009). Symptom complaints following combat-related traumatic brain injury: Relationship to traumatic brain injury severity and posttraumatic stress disorder. *Journal of the International Neuropsychological Society, 16* (01), 194–199.

Bilbul, M., & Schipper, H. M. (2011). Risk profiles of Alzheimer disease. *Canadian Journal of Neurological Sciences/Journal Canadien des Sciences Neurologiques, 38*(04), 580–592.

Blanchard, E. B., Hickling, E. J., Taylor, A. E., Forneris, C. A., Loos, W., & Jaccard, J. (1995). Effects of varying scoring rules of the Clinician-Administered PTSD Scale (CAPS) for the diagnosis of post-traumatic stress disorder in motor vehicle accident victims. *Behaviour Research and Therapy, 33*(4), 471–475.

Blanchard, E. B., Hickling, E. J., Taylor, A. E., Loos, W. R., Forneris, C. A., & Jaccard, J. (1996). Who develops PTSD from motor vehicle accidents? *Behaviour Research and Therapy, 34*(1), 1–10.

Bombardier, C. H., Fann, J. R., Temkin, N., Esselman, P. C., Pelzer, E., Keough, M., et al. (2006). Posttraumatic stress disorder symptoms during the first six months after traumatic brain injury. *The Journal of Neuropsychiatry and Clinical Neurosciences, 18*(4), 501–508.

Butcher, J. N., Graham, J. R., Ben-Porath, Y. S., Tellegen, A., & Dahlstrom, W. G. (1989). *Manual for the administration, scoring, and interpretation: Minnesota multiphasic personality inventory-2 (MMPI-2)*. Minnesota: University of Minnesota Press Minneapolis.

Bremner, J. D., Krystal, J. H., Southwick, S. M., & Charney, D. S. (1995). Functional neuroanatomical correlates of the effects of stress on memory. *Journal of Traumatic Stress, 8* (4), 527–553.

© The Author(s) 2016

C.J. Golden et al., *The Intercorrelation of Traumatic Brain Injury and PTSD in Neuropsychological Evaluations*, SpringerBriefs in Behavioral Criminology, DOI 10.1007/978-3-319-47033-7

Bruns, J. J., & Jagoda, A. S. (2009). Mild traumatic brain injury. *Mount Sinai Journal of Medicine: A Journal of Translational and Personalized Medicine, 76*(2), 129–137.

Bryant, R. A., & Harvey, A. G. (1998). Relationship between acute stress disorder and posttraumatic stress disorder following mild traumatic brain injury. *American Journal of Psychiatry, 155*, 625–629.

Bryant, R. A., Marosszeky, J. E., Crooks, J., & Gurka, J. A. (2000). Posttraumatic stress disorder after severe traumatic brain injury. *American Journal of Psychiatry, 157*, 629–631.

Butcher, J., Graham, J., Ben-Porath, Y, Tellegen, A, & Dhalstrom, W. G. (2001). *MMPI-2: Minnesota multiphasic personality inventory-2: Manual for administration, scoring, and interpretation.* University of Minnesota Press.

Carrion, V. G., Garrett, A., Menon, V., Weems, C. F., & Reiss, A. L. (2008). Posttraumatic stress symptoms and brain function during a response-inhibition task: An fMRI study in youth. *Depression and Anxiety, 25*(6), 514–526.

Church, D., & Palmer-Hoffman, J. (2014). TBI symptoms improve after PTSD remediation with emotional freedom techniques. *Traumatology, 20*(3), 172.

Collins, M. W., Iverson, G. L., Lovell, M. R., McKeag, D. B., Norwig, J., & Maroon, J. (2003). On-field predictors of neuropsychological and symptom deficit following sports-related concussion. *Clinical Journal of Sport Medicine, 13*(4), 222–229.

Conners, C. K. (2014). *Conners continuous performance test 3rd edition (Conners CPT 3) & conners continuous auditory test of attention (Conners CATA)—technical manual.* New York, Toronto: MHS.

Coronado, V. G., McGuire, L. C., Sarmiento, K., Bell, J., Lionbarger, M. R., Jones, C. D., et al. (2012). Trends in traumatic brain injury in the US and the public health response: 1995–2009. *Journal of safety research, 43*(4), 299–307.

Deb, S., Lyons, I., Koutzoukis, C., Ali, I., & McCarthy, G. (1999). Rate of psychiatric illness 1 year after traumatic brain injury. *American Journal of Psychiatry, 156*(3), 374–378.

DePalma, R. G., Burris, D. G., Champion, H. R., & Hodgson, M. J. (2005). Blast injuries. *New England Journal of Medicine, 352*(13), 1335–1342.

Elder, G. A., Mitsis, E. M., Ahlers, S. T., & Cristian, A. (2010). Blast-induced mild traumatic brain injury. *Psychiatric Clinics of North America, 33*(4), 757–781.

Exner Jr, J. E. (2002). *The Rorschach: a comprehensive system, vol. 1. Basic foundations and principles of interpretation,* 4th Ed. Wiley.

Federoff, J. P., Starkstein, S. E., Forrester, A. W., Geisler, F. H., Jorge, R. E., Arndt, S. V., et al. (1992). Depression in patients with acute traumatic brain injury. *American Journal of Psychiatry, 149*, 918–923.

Fann, J. R., Katon, W. J., Uomoto, J. M., & Esselman, P. C. (1995). Psychiatric disorders and functional disability in outpatients with traumatic brain injuries. *American Journal of Psychiatry, 152*, 1493–1499.

Faul, M., & Coronado, V. (2014). Epidemiology of traumatic brain injury. *Handbook of clinical neurology, 127*, 3–13.

Glasser, R. (2007). A shock wave of brain injuries. *The Washington Post, 8.*

Golden, C. J. (1976). The identification of brain damage by an abbreviated form of the Halstead-Reitan neuropsychological battery. *Journal of Clinical Psychology, 32*(4), 821–826.

Golden, C. J., Espe-Pfeifer, P., & Wachsler-Felder, J. (2000). *Neuropsychological interpretation of objective psychological tests.* Springer.

Golden, C. J., & Freshwater, S. M. (2002). *The Stroop color and word test: A manual for clinical and experimental uses.* Illinois: Stoeling Co.

Golden, C. J., Zillmer, E., & Spiers, M. (1992). *Neuropsychological assessment and intervention.* Charles C Thomas, Publisher.

Golden, C. J., & Lashley, L. (2014). *Forensic neuropsychological evaluation of the violent offender.* Springer.

Graham, J. R. (2011). *MMPI-2: Assessing personality and psychopathology* (5th ed.). New York: Oxford University Press.

Harvey, A. G., & Bryant, R. A. (1998). The relationship between acute stress disorder and posttraumatic stress disorder: A prospective evaluation of motor vehicle accident survivors. *Journal of Consulting and Clinical Psychology, 66*(3), 507.

Harvey, A. G., & Bryant, R. A. (2000). Memory for acute stress disorder symptoms: A two-year prospective study. *The Journal of Nervous and Mental Disease, 188*(9), 602–607.

Heaton, R. K., Chelune, G. J., Talley, J. L., Kay, G. G., & Curtiss, G. (1993). *Wisconsin card sorting test manual revised and expanded*. Lutz, FL: Psychological Assessment Resources.

Hibbard, M. R., Uysal, S., Kepler, K., Bogdany, J., & Silver, J. (1998). Axis I psychopathology in individuals with traumatic brain injury. *The Journal of Head Trauma Rehabilitation, 13*(4), 24–39.

Hickling, E. J., Gillen, R., Blanchard, E. B., Buckley, T., & Taylor, A. (1998). Traumatic brain injury and posttraumatic stress disorder: A preliminary investigation of neuropsychological test results in PTSD secondary to motor vehicle accidents. *Brain Injury, 12*(4), 265–274.

Hoge, C. W., McGurk, D., Thomas, J. L., Cox, A. L., Engel, C. C., & Castro, C. A. (2008). Mild traumatic brain injury in US soldiers returning from Iraq. *New England Journal of Medicine, 358*(5), 453–463.

Hoofien, D., Gilboa, A., Vakil, E., & Donovick, P. J. (2001). Traumatic brain injury (tbi) 10–20 years later: A comprehensive outcome study of psychiatric symptomatology, cognitive abilities and psychosocial functioning. *Brain Injury, 15*(3), 189–209.

Hyder, A. A., Wunderlich, C. A., Puvanachandra, P., Gururaj, G., & Kobusingye, O. C. (2007). The impact of traumatic brain injuries: A global perspective. *NeuroRehabilitation-An Interdisciplinary Journal, 22*(5), 341–354.

Iverson, G. L., & Lange, R. T. (2011). Mild traumatic brain injury. In *The little black book of neuropsychology* (pp. 697–719). Springer: USA.

Iverson, G. L., Lovell, M. R., & Smith, S. S. (2000). Does brief loss of consciousness affect cognitive functioning after mild head injury? *Archives of Clinical Neuropsychology, 15*(7), 643–648.

Jellinger, K. A. (2004). Head injury and dementia. *Current Opinion in Neurology, 17*(6), 719–723.

Johnsen, G. E., & Asbjørnsen, A. E. (2008). Consistent impaired verbal memory in PTSD: A meta-analysis. *Journal of Affective Disorders, 111*(1), 74–82.

Johnson, V. E., Stewart, W., & Smith, D. H. (2010). Traumatic brain injury and amyloid-β pathology: A link to Alzheimer's disease? *Nature Reviews Neuroscience, 11*(5), 361–370.

Jorge, R. E., Robinson, R. G., Arndt, S. V., Starkstein, S. E., Forrester, A. W., & Geisler, F. (1993). Depression following traumatic brain injury: A 1 year longitudinal study. *Journal of Affective Disorders, 27*(4), 233–243.

Kennedy, J. E., Cullen, M. A., Amador, R. R., Huey, J. C., & Leal, F. O. (2010). Symptoms in military service members after blast mTBI with and without associated injuries. *NeuroRehabilitation, 26*(3), 191–197.

Kessler, R. C., Sonnega, A., Bromet, E., Hughes, M., & Nelson, C. B. (1995). Posttraumatic stress disorder in the National Comorbidity Survey. *Archives of General Psychiatry, 52*(12), 1048–1060.

Koponen, S., Taiminen, T., Portin, R., Himanen, L., Isoniemi, H., Heinonen, H., et al. (2002). Axis I and II psychiatric disorders after traumatic brain injury: A 30-year follow-up study. *American Journal of Psychiatry, 159*, 1315–1321.

Lange, R. T., Brickell, T. A., Kennedy, J. E., Bailie, J. M., Sills, C., Asmussen, S., et al. (2014). Factors influencing postconcussion and posttraumatic stress symptom reporting following military-related concurrent polytrauma and traumatic brain injury. *Archives of Clinical Neuropsychology, 29*, 329–347.

Langlois, J. A., Rutland-Brown, W., & Wald, M. M. (2006). The epidemiology and impact of traumatic brain injury: A brief overview. *The Journal of Head Trauma Rehabilitation, 21*(5), 375–378.

Leininger, B. E., Gramling, S. E., Farrell, A. D., Kreutzer, J. S., & Peck, E. A. (1990). Neuropsychological deficits in symptomatic minor head injury patients after concussion and mild concussion. *Journal of Neurology, Neurosurgery & Psychiatry, 53*(4), 293–296.

Lippa, S. M., Pastorek, N. J., Benge, J. F., & Thornton, G. M. (2010). Postconcussive symptoms after blast and nonblast-related mild traumatic brain injuries in Afghanistan and Iraq war veterans. *Journal of the International Neuropsychological Society, 16*(5), 856–866.

Lovell, M. R., Iverson, G. L., Collins, M. W., McKeag, D., & Maroon, J. C. (1999). Does loss of consciousness predict neuropsychological decrements after concussion? *Clinical Journal of Sport Medicine, 9*(4), 193–198.

Lye, T. C., & Shores, E. A. (2000). Traumatic brain injury as a risk factor for Alzheimer's disease: A review. *Neuropsychology Review, 10*(2), 115–129.

Lyons, J. A., & Wheeler-Cox, T. (1999). MMPI, MMPI-2 and PTSD: Overview of scores, scales, and profiles. *Journal of Traumatic Stress, 12*(1), 175–183.

Mather, F. J., Tate, R. L., & Hannan, T. J. (2003). Post-traumatic stress disorder in children following road traffic accidents: A comparison of those with and without mild traumatic brain injury. *Brain Injury, 17*(12), 1077–1087.

Matthews, S. C., Strigo, I. A., Simmons, A. N., O'Connell, R. M., Reinhardt, L. E., & Moseley, S. A. (2011). A multimodal imaging study in U.S. veterans of operations Iraqi and enduring freedom with and without major depression after blast-related concussion. *Neuroimage, 54*, S69–S75.

McAllister, T. W., Flashman, L. A., McDonald, B. C., & Saykin, A. J. (2006). Mechanisms of working memory dysfunction after mild and moderate TBI: Evidence from functional MRI and neurogenetics. *Journal of Neurotrauma, 23*(10), 1450–1467.

McCrea, M., Kelly, J. P., Randolph, C., Cisler, R., & Berger, L. (2002). Immediate neurocognitive effects of concussion. *Neurosurgery, 50*(5), 1032–1042.

McMillan, T. M. (1991). Post traumatic stress disorder and severe head injury. *The British Journal of Psychiatry, 159*, 431–433.

McMillan, T. M., Williams, W. H., & Bryant, R. (2003). Post-traumatic stress disorder and traumatic brain injury: A review of causal mechanisms, assessment, and treatment. *Neuropsychological Rehabilitation, 13*(1–2), 149–164.

Millon, T., Millon, C., Davis, R. D., & Grossman, S. (2009). *Millon clinical multiaxial inventory-III (MCMI-III): Manual.* Pearson/PsychCorp.

Murray, C. J., & Lopez, A. D. (1996). Evidence-based health policy–lessons from the global burden of disease study. *Science, 274*(5288), 740.

Okie, S. (2005). Traumatic brain injury in war zone. *The New England Journal of Medicine, 352* (20), 2043–2046.

Qureshi, S. U., Kimbrell, T., Pyne, J. M., Magruder, K. M., Hudson, T. J., & Petersen, N. J. (2010). Greater prevalence and incidence of dementia in older veterans with posttraumatic stress disorder. *Journal of the American Geriatrics Society, 58*(9), 1627–1633.

Rauch, S. L., Shin, L. M., & Phelps, E. A. (2006). Neurocircuitry models of posttraumatic stress disorder and extinction: Human neuroimaging research—past, present, and future. *Biological psychiatry, 60*(4), 376–382.

Rogers, R., Sewell, K. W., & Gillard, N. D. (2010). *SIRS-2: Structured interview of reported symptoms: Professional manual.* Psychological Assessment Resources, Incorporated.

Sbordone, R. J., & Liter, J. C. (1995). Mild traumatic brain injury does not produce post-traumatic stress disorder. *Brain Injury, 9*(4), 405–412.

Schneiderman, A. I., Braver, E. R., & Kang, H. K. (2008). Understanding sequelae of injury mechanisms and mild traumatic brain injury incurred during the conflicts in Iraq and Afghanistan: Persistent postconcussive symptoms and posttraumatic stress disorder. *American Journal of Epidemiology, 167*(12), 1446–1452.

Shu, I. W., Onton, J. A., Prabhakar, N., O'Connell, R. M., Simmons, A. N., & Matthews, S. C. (2014). Combat veterans with PTSD after mild TBI exhibit greater ERPs from posterior-medial cortical areas while appraising facial features. *Journal of Affective Disorders, 155*, 234–240.

Simmons, A. N., & Matthews, S. C. (2012). Neural circuitry of PTSD with or without mild traumatic brain injury: A meta-analysis. *Neuropharmacology, 62*(2), 598–606.

Stein, M. B., & McAllister, T. W. (2009). Exploring the convergence of posttraumatic stress disorder and mild traumatic brain injury. *American Journal of Psychiatry, 166*(7), 768–776.

Sundin, J., Fear, N. T., Iversen, A., Rona, R. J., & Wessely, S. (2010). PTSD after deployment to Iraq: Conflicting rates, conflicting claims. *Psychological Medicine, 40*(3), 367–382.

Swick, D., Honzel, N., Larsen, J., Ashley, V., & Justus, T. (2012). Impaired response inhibition in veterans with post-traumatic stress disorder and mild traumatic brain injury. *Journal of the International Neuropsychological Society, 18*(5), 917–926.

Tanielian, T. L., & Jaycox, L. (Eds.). (2008). *Invisible wounds of war: Psychological and cognitive injuries, their consequences, and services to assist recovery* (vol. 1). Rand Corporation.

Tombaugh, T. N. (1996). *Test of memory malingering: M.* New York/Toronto: MHS.

Trudeau, D. L., Anderson, J., Hansen, L. M., Shagalov, D. N., Schmoller, J., Nugent, S., et al. (1998). Findings of mild traumatic brain injury in combat veterans with PTSD and a history of blast concussion. *The Journal of Neuropsychiatry and Clinical Neurosciences., 10*, 308–313.

Ursano, R. J., Fullerton, C. S., Epstein, R. S., Crowley, B., Vance, K., Kao, T. C., et al. (1999). Peritraumatic dissociation and posttraumatic stress disorder following motor vehicle accidents. *American Journal of Psychiatry, 156*(11), 1808–1810.

Van Reekum, R., Bolago, I., Finlayson, M. A. J., Garner, S., & Links, P. S. (1996). Psychiatric disorders after traumatic brain injury. *Brain Injury, 10*(5), 319–328.

Van Reekum, R., Cohen, T., & Wong, J. (2000). Can traumatic brain injury cause psychiatric disorders? *The Journal of Neuropsychiatry and Clinical neurosciences, 12*(3), 316–327.

Varney, N. R., Matrzke, J. S., & Roberts, R. J. (1987). Major depression in patients with closed head injury. *Neuropsychology, 1*, 7–9.

Vasterling, J. J., Brailey, K., Constans, J. I., & Sutker, P. B. (1998). Attention and memory dysfunction in posttraumatic stress disorder. *Neuropsychology, 12*(1), 125.

Warden, D. (2006). Military TBI during the Iraq and Afghanistan wars. *The Journal of Head Trauma Rehabilitation, 21*(5), 398–402.

Weiner, M. W., Veitch, D. P., Hayes, J., Neylan, T., Grafman, J., Aisen, P. S., et al. (2014). Effects of traumatic brain injury and posttraumatic stress disorder on Alzheimer's disease in veterans, using the Alzheimer's disease neuroimaging initiative. *Alzheimer's & Dementia, 10*(3), S226–S235.

Wechsler, D. (2008). *WAIS-IV manual.* New York: The Psychological Corporation.

Wechsler, D. (2009). *WMS-IV: Administration and scoring manual.* San Antonio, TX: The Psychological Corporation.

Wechsler, D. (2009). *WMS-IV: Wechsler memory scale-technical and interpretive manual.* San Antonio, TX: Pearson.

Williams, W. H., Evans, J. J., Wilson, B. A., & Needham, P. (2002). Brief report: Prevalence of post-traumatic stress disorder symptoms after severe traumatic brain injury in a representative community sample. *Brain Injury, 16*(8), 673–679.

Yaffe, K., Vittinghoff, E., Lindquist, K., Barnes, D., Covinsky, K. E., Neylan, T., et al. (2010). Posttraumatic stress disorder and risk of dementia among US veterans. *Archives of General Psychiatry, 67*(6), 608–613.

Yeh, P. H., Wang, B., Oakes, T. R., French, L. M., Pan, H., Graner, J., et al. (2014). Postconcussional disorder and PTSD symptoms of military-related traumatic brain injury associated with compromised neurocircuitry. *Human Brain Mapping, 35*(6), 2652–2673.

Yehuda, R., Golier, J. A., Halligan, S. L., & Harvey, P. D. (2004). Learning and memory in Holocaust survivors with posttraumatic stress disorder. *Biological Psychiatry, 55*(3), 291–295.

Yurgil, K. A., Barkauskas, D. A., Vasterling, J. J., Nievergelt, C. M., Larson, G. E., Schork, N. J., et al. (2014). Association between traumatic brain injury and risk of posttraumatic stress disorder in active-duty Marines. *JAMA Psychiatry, 71*(2), 149–157.

Zillmer, E. A., Spiers, M. V. (2001). *Principles of neuropsychology.* Wadsworth Publishing Company.